The Complete Vegetarian Side Dish Cookbook

Easy And Delicious Side Dish Vegetarian Recipes

Adam Denton

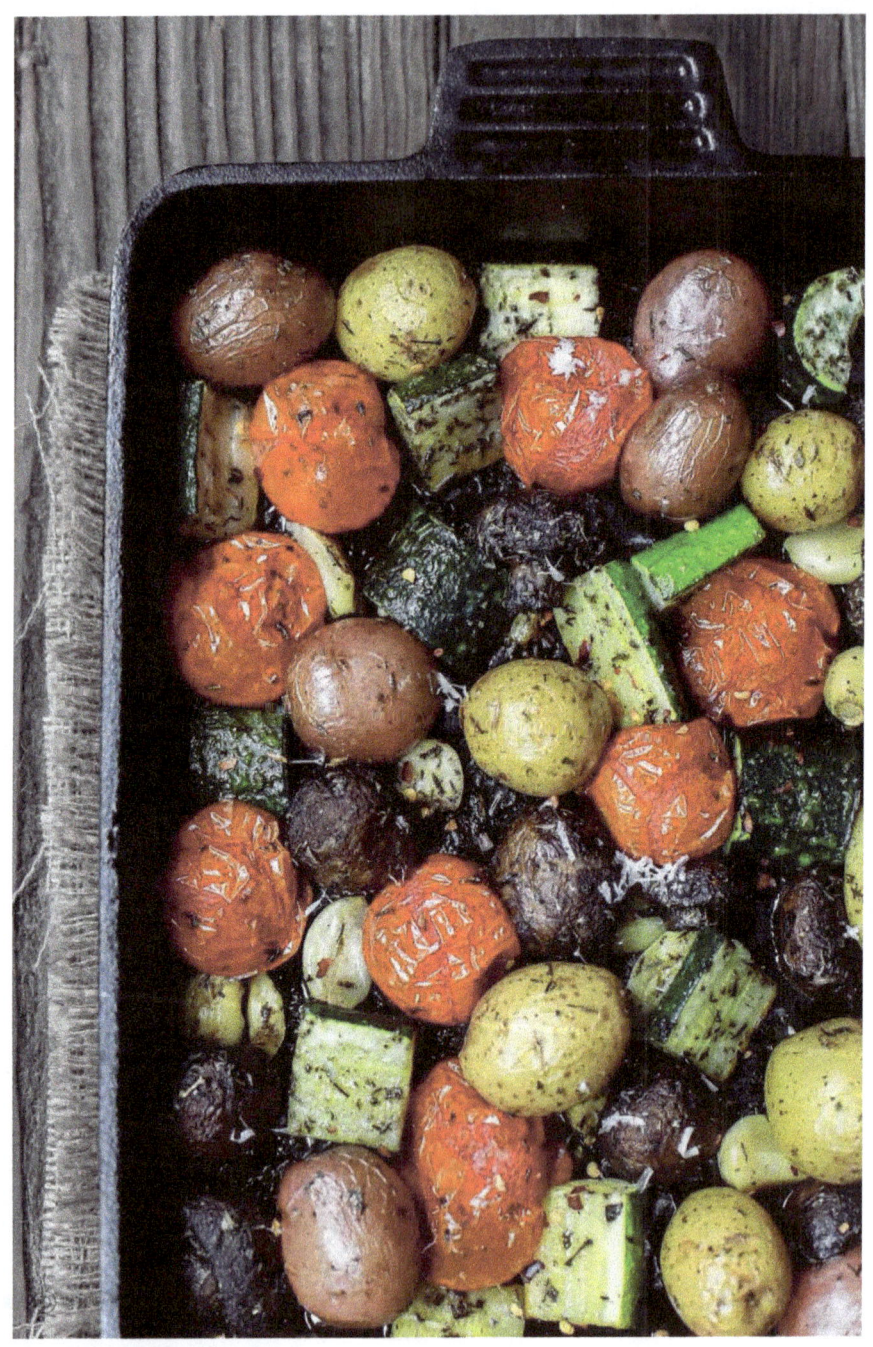

© **Copyright 2020 - All rights reserved.**

The content contained within this book may not be reproduced, duplicated or transmitted without direct written permission from the author or the publisher.

Under no circumstances will any blame or legal responsibility be held against the publisher, or author, for any damages, reparation, or monetary loss due to the information contained within this book. Either directly or indirectly.

Legal Notice:

This book is copyright protected. This book is only for personal use. You cannot amend, distribute, sell, use, quote or paraphrase any part, or the content within this book, without the consent of the author or publisher.

Disclaimer Notice:

Please note the information contained within this document is for educational and entertainment purposes only. All effort has been executed to present accurate, up to date, and reliable, complete information. No warranties of any kind are declared or implied. Readers acknowledge that the author is not engaging in the rendering of legal, financial, medical or professional advice. The content within this book has been derived from various sources. Please consult a licensed professional before attempting any techniques outlined in this book.

By reading this document, the reader agrees that under no circumstances is the author responsible for any losses, direct or indirect, which are incurred as a result of the use of information contained within this document, including, but not limited to, — errors, omissions, or inaccuracies.

Table of contents

Masala Brown, Green and Pardina Lentils 7

Swiss Chard and White Bean Stew 9

Faro and Kidney Bean Chili 11

Grilled Zucchini and Cremini Mushrooms with Balsamic Glaze 13

Grilled Zucchini and Red Onions in Ranch Dressing 15

Grilled Marinated Eggplant and Zucchini 17

Grilled Cauliflower and Brussel Sprouts 19

Grilled Eggplant, Zucchini and Corn 21

Grilled Portobello and Eggplant 23

Grilled Japanese Eggplant and Shitake Mushroom 25

Broccoli Florets Marinade 27

Grilled Portobello Asparagus and Pineapple 29

Brussel Sprouts and Endives 31

Grilled Green Bean and Microgreens in Balsamic Vinaigrette 33

Grilled Broccolini and Turnip Greens 35

Grilled Green Cabbage in Apple Cider Vinaigrette 37

Grilled Parsnip and Rutabaga 39

Grilled Carrot, Turnip and Water Chestnuts with Balsamic Glaze 41

Grilled beetroots and Green Beans 43

Grilles Turnips Broccolini and Water Chestnuts with Honey Apple Cider Glaze 44

Grilled Eggplant & Beetroot with Assorted Bell Peppers 45

Grilled Water Chestnuts Zucchini and Endives 47

Grilled Collard Greens Portobello and Asparagus 49

Grilled Ruttabaga and Swiss Chard 51

Grilled Green Beans and Eggplants 53

Grilled Collard Greens and Brussel Sprouts 55

Grilled Swiss Chard and Asparagus 57

Grilled Endives and Edamame Beans 59

Grilled Water Chestnuts and Cabbage 61

Grilled Okra and Waterchestnuts 63

Grilled Turnip Greens and Broccolini 65

Grilled Parsnip and Microgreens 67

Grilled Carrot, Parsnip and Endives 69

Grilled Cauliflower and Baby Corn 71

Grilled Baby Carrots and Beetroots 73

Grilled Microgreens and Beetroots 75

Grilled Rutabaga Pineapple and Artichoke Hearts 77

Simple Grilled Water Chestnuts and Cauliflower Florets 79

Grilled Baby Corn, Water Chestnuts and Eggplant 81

Grilled Broccolini Beetroots and Portobello Mushroom 83

Grilled Baby Carrots and Baby Carrots 85

Grilled Turnip Greens 87

Grilled Broccolini Florets and Summer Squash 89

Grilled Winter Squash and Eggplant 91

Grilled Zucchini and Green Bell Peppers 93

Grilled Zucchini & Butternut Squash 95

Grilled Baby Corn Zucchini and Beetroots...97

Grilled Summer Squash and Carrots.. 99

Grilled Edamame Beans and Zucchini 101

Grilled Okra and Mustard Greens 103

Grilled Beetroots & Kale..105

Grilled Edamame Beans and Summer Squash 107

Masala Brown, Green and Pardina Lentils

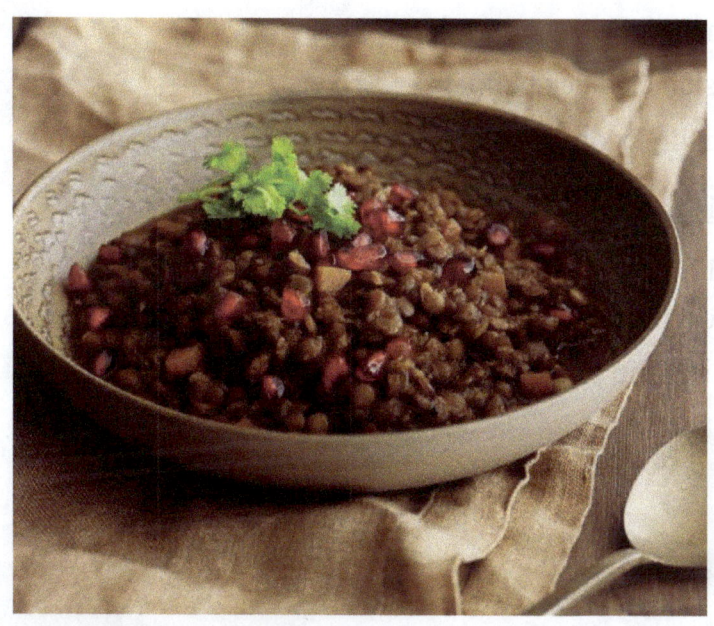

Ingredients

1 red onion, chopped

5 cloves garlic, minced

1 tablespoon minced fresh ginger, or 1 teaspoon ground ginger powder

2¼ cups brown, green or pardina lentils

4 cups vegetable broth

1 15-ounce can diced San Marzano tomatoes, with their juices

¼ cup tomato paste

2 teaspoons tamarind paste (optional, adds a hint of tartness)

1 teaspoon honey

¾ teaspoon sea salt

1½ teaspoon garam masala

A few shakes black pepper

1 cup light coconut milk

Side dish:

Rice, quinoa, or another whole grain and fresh herbs

Put everything except for the coconut milk and side dish ingredients in the slow cooker.

Directions:

Combine thoroughly and cook on high for 3 and a half hours or on low for 6 hours. In the last hour, check if more liquid needs to be added. When the lentils become more tender, add the coconut milk. Add this to the rice, quinoa and fresh herbs.

Swiss Chard and White Bean Stew

Ingredients

2 pounds white beans (sorted and rinsed)
2 large carrots, peeled and diced
3 large celery stalks, diced
1 red onion, diced
6 cloves garlic, minced or chopped
1 bay leaf
1 tsp. each: dried rosemary, thyme, oregano
11 cups water
2 Tbsp. salt
Ground black pepper, to taste
1 large can (28 ounces) diced tomatoes
5-6 cups chopped
Swiss chard & kale
Rice, polenta, or bread for serving

Directions:

Combine beans, carrots, celery, onions, garlic, bay leaf and dried herbs. Add the water. Cook on high heat for 3 ½ hours, or low heat for 9 hours. Remove lid from slow cooker and season with salt and pepper Add diced tomatoes. Cook for another 1 hour and 15 min. or until beans get very soft. Garnish with the chopped greens. Serve with cooked rice, polenta, or with bread.

Faro and Kidney Bean Chili

Ingredients:

1 cup uncooked faro

1 medium red or yellow onion, peeled and diced

8 cloves of garlic, minced

1 chipotle chili in adobo sauce, chopped

2 (15 ounce) cans dark red kidney beans, rinsed and drained (**see below for substitution ideas)

2 (15 ounce) cans tomato sauce

2 (14 ounce) cans diced tomatoes

1 (15 ounce) can light red kidney beans, rinsed and drained

1 (4 ounce) can chopped red chilies

4 cups vegetable broth

1 cup beer (or you can just add extra vegetable broth)

2 Tablespoons chili powder

1 tablespoon ground cumin

1 teaspoon sea salt

1 teaspoon honey

1/2 teaspoon black pepper

Directions:

Combine all of the ingredients in a slow cooker and stir thoroughly. Cook on high for 3 ½ hours or on low heat for 7 hours until the beans are soft. Taste, and add more salt and pepper if necessary. Garnish with toppings. Refrigerate for 3 days or freeze for 3 months.

Grilled Zucchini and Cremini Mushrooms with Balsamic Glaze

Ingredients

3 yellow bell peppers, seeded and halved

3 summer squash (about 1 pound total), sliced lengthwise into 1/2-inch-thick rectangles

3 zucchini (about 12 ounces total), sliced lengthwise into 1/2-inch- thick rectangles

3 eggplant (12 ounces total), sliced lengthwise into 1/2-inch-thick rectangles

12 cremini mushrooms

1 bunch (1-pound) asparagus, trimmed 12 green onions, roots cut off

6 tablespoons olive oil

Salt and freshly ground black pepper

3 tablespoons balsamic vinegar

4 garlic cloves, minced

1 teaspoon chopped fresh parsley leaves

1 teaspoon chopped fresh basil leaves

1/2 teaspoon finely chopped fresh rosemary leaves

Directions:

Preheat your grill for medium-high heat Lightly brush the vegetables with 1/4 cup of the oil Season the vegetables with salt and pepper. Working in batches, grill them until tender. Combine the 2 Tablespoons of oil, balsamic vinegar, garlic, parsley, basil, and rosemary in a bowl. Season with salt and pepper. Drizzle the vinaigrette over the vegetables.

Grilled Zucchini and Red Onions in Ranch Dressing

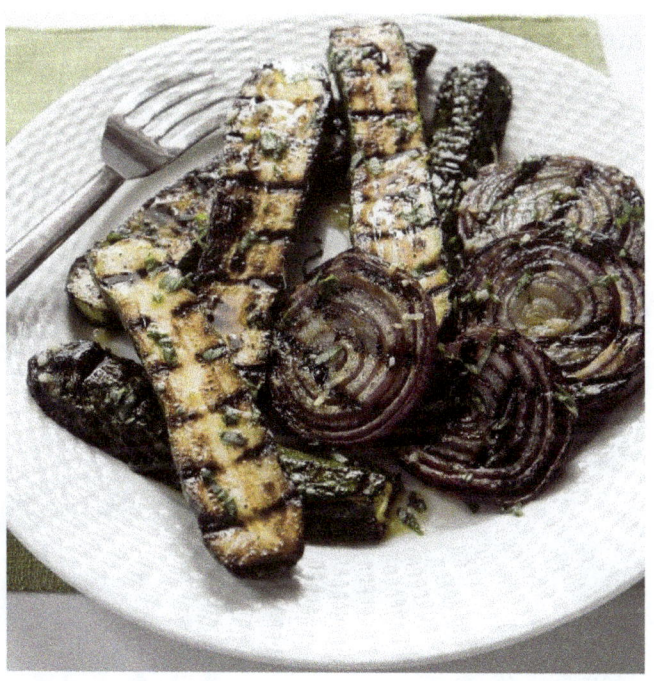

Ingredients

2 large zucchini , cut lengthwise into ½ inch slabs

2 large red onions, cut into ½ inch rings but don't separate into individual rings

2 tbsp. extra virgin olive oil

2 tbsp. ranch dressing mix

Directions:

Lightly brush each side of the vegetables with olive oil. Season with the ranch dressing mix Grill over 4 minutes over medium heat or until tender.

Grilled Marinated Eggplant and Zucchini

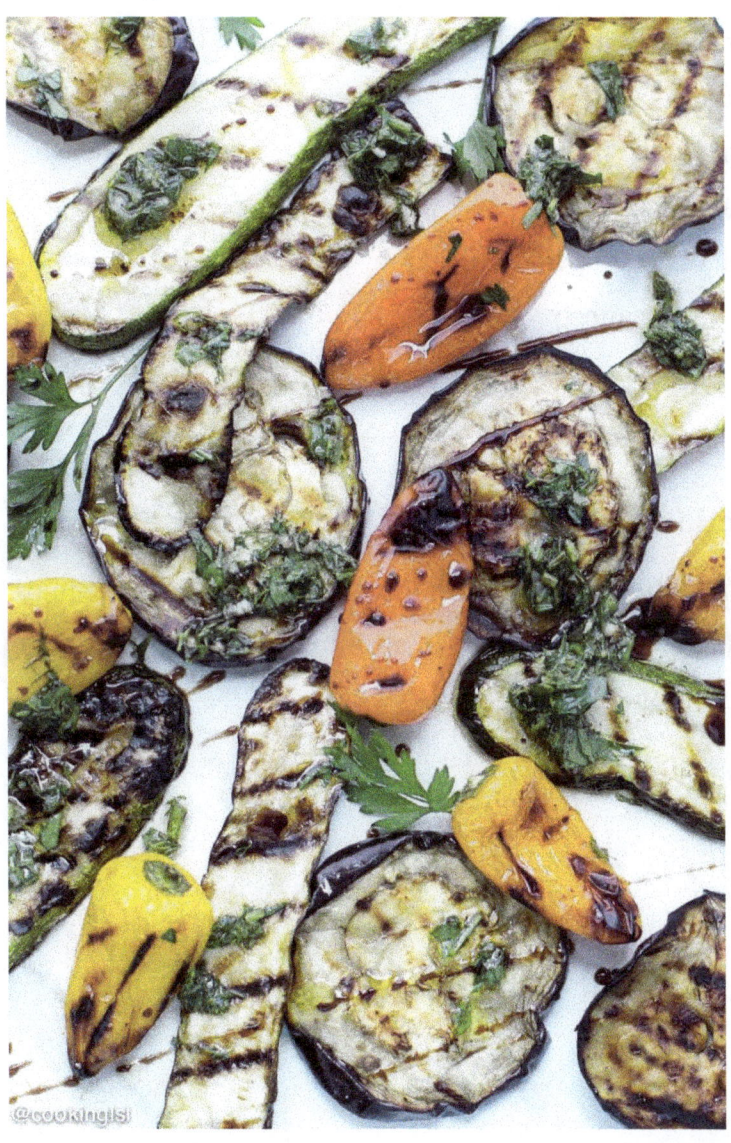

Ingredients

2 large Eggplants, cut lengthwise and cut in half

2 large Zucchinis, cut lengthwise and cut in half Marinade ingredients:

6 tbsp. extra virgin olive oil

Sea salt, to taste

3 tbsp. distilled white vinegar

1 tsp. pesto sauce

Directions:

Marinate the vegetable with the dressing or Marinade ingredients for 15 to 30 min. Grill for 4 minutes over medium heat or until the vegetable becomes tender.

Grilled Cauliflower and Brussel Sprouts

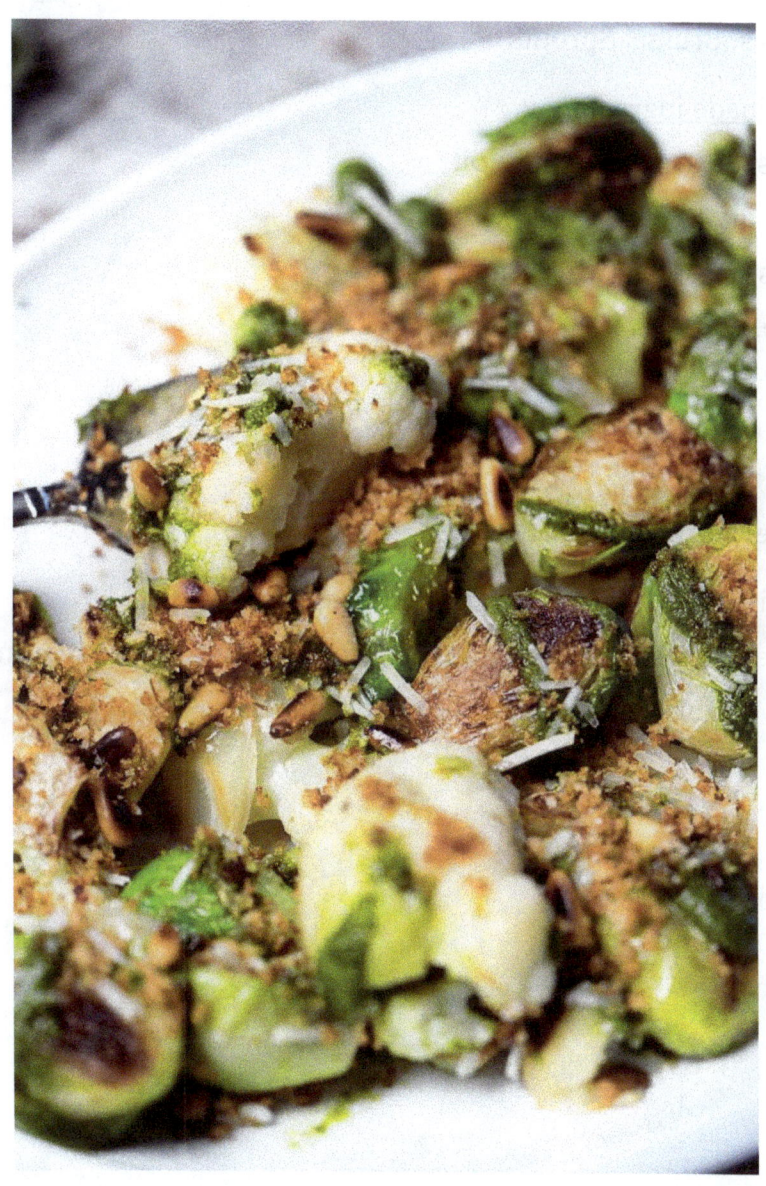

Ingredients

10 Cauliflower florets

10 pcs. Brussel Sprouts

Marinade ingredients:

6 tbsp. extra virgin olive oil

Sea salt, to taste

3 tbsp. distilled white vinegar

1 tsp. mayonnaise

Directions:

Marinate the vegetable with the dressing or Marinade ingredients for 15 to 30 min. Grill for 4 minutes over medium heat or until the vegetable becomes tender.

Grilled Eggplant, Zucchini and Corn

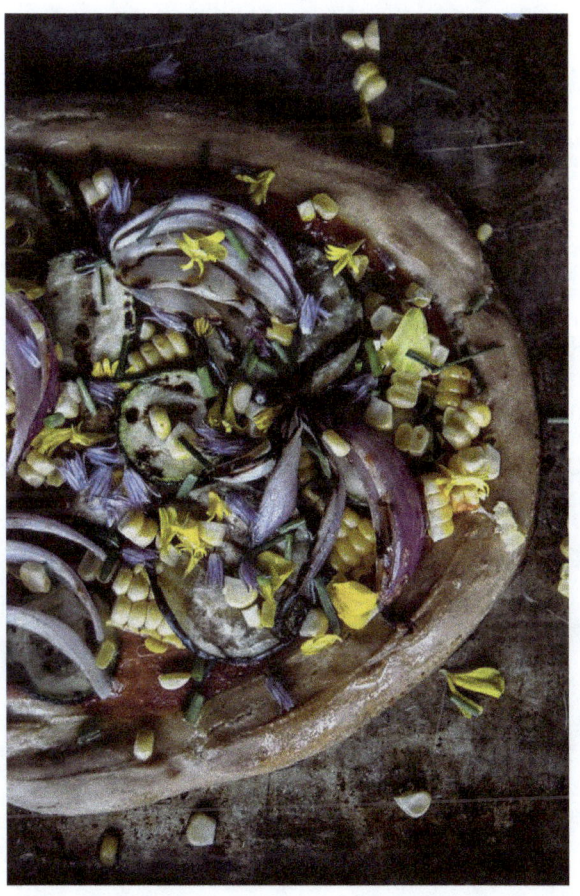

Ingredients

2 large Eggplants, cut lengthwise and cut in half

2 large Zucchinis, cut lengthwise and cut in half

2 Corns, cut lengthwise

Marinade ingredients:

6 tbsp. extra virgin olive oil

Sea salt, to taste

3 tbsp. distilled white vinegar

1 tsp. mayonnaise

Directions:

Marinate the vegetable with the dressing or Marinade ingredients for 15 to 30 min. Grill for 4 minutes over medium heat or until the vegetable becomes tender.

Grilled Portobello and Eggplant

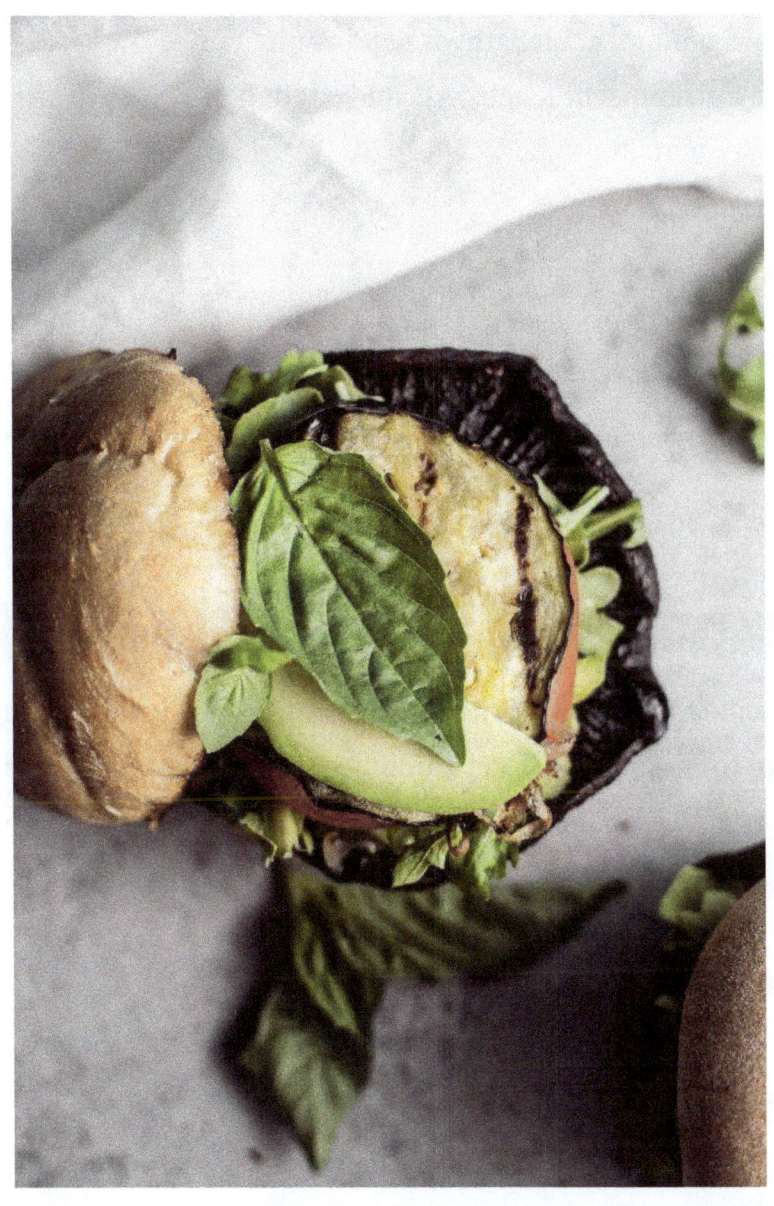

Ingredients

3 pcs. Portobello, rinsed and drained

2 pcs. Eggplant, cut lengthwise and cut in half

2 pcs. Zucchini, cut lengthwise and cut in half

6 pcs. Asparagus

<u>Marinade ingredients:</u>

6 tbsp. extra virgin olive oil

Sea salt, to taste

3 tbsp. distilled white vinegar

1 tsp. English mustard

Directions:

Marinate the vegetable with the dressing or Marinade ingredients for 15 to 30 min. Grill for 4 minutes over medium heat or until the vegetable becomes tender.

Grilled Japanese Eggplant and Shitake Mushroom

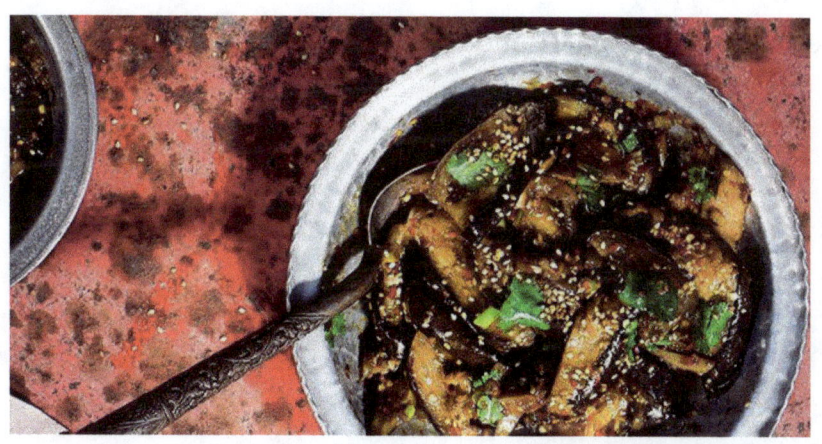

Ingredients

Corns, cut lengthwise

2 pcs. Japanese Eggplant, cut lengthwise and cut in half

3 Shitake Mushrooms, rinsed and drained

Dressing Ingredients

6 tbsp. olive oil

Sea salt, to taste

3 tbsp. white wine vinegar

1 tsp. Egg-free mayonnaise

Directions:

Marinate the vegetable with the dressing or Marinade ingredients for 15 to 30 min. Grill for 4 minutes over medium heat or until the vegetable becomes tender.

Broccoli Florets Marinade

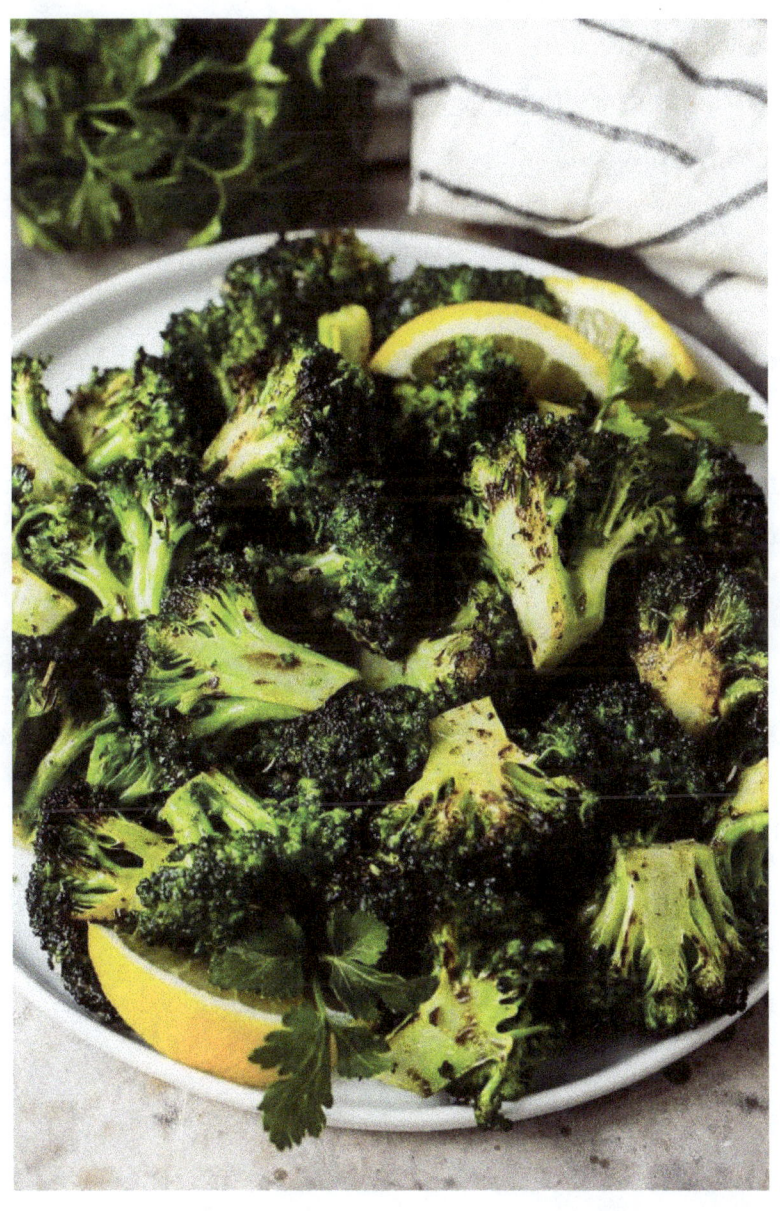

Ingredients:

6 tbsp. extra virgin olive oil

Sea salt, to taste

3 tbsp. distilled white vinegar

1 tsp. mayonnaise

Directions:

Marinate the vegetable with the dressing or Marinade ingredients for 15 to 30 min. Grill for 4 minutes over medium heat or until the vegetable becomes tender.

Grilled Portobello Asparagus and Pineapple

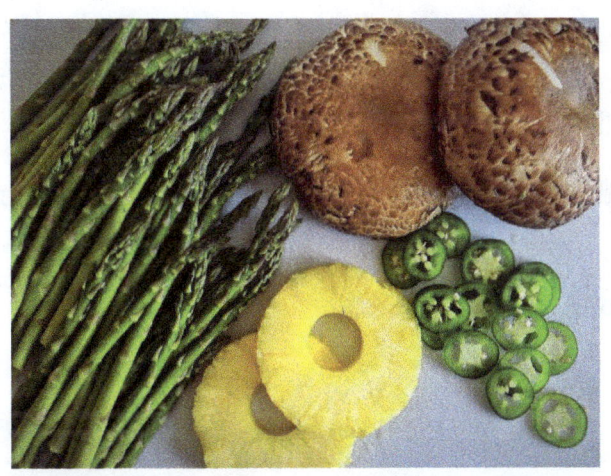

Ingredients

3 pcs. Portobello, rinsed and drained

2 pcs. Eggplant, cut lengthwise and cut in half

2 pcs. Zucchini, cut lengthwise and cut in half

6 pcs. Asparagus

1 medium Pineapple, cut into 1/2 inch slices

10 Green Beans

<u>Dressing Ingredients</u>

6 tbsp. extra virgin olive oil

Sea salt, to taste

3 tbsp. apple cider vinegar

1 tbsp. honey

1 tsp. mayonnaise

Directions:

Marinate the vegetable with the dressing or Marinade ingredients for 15 to 30 min. Grill for 4 minutes over medium heat or until the vegetable becomes tender.

Brussel Sprouts and Endives

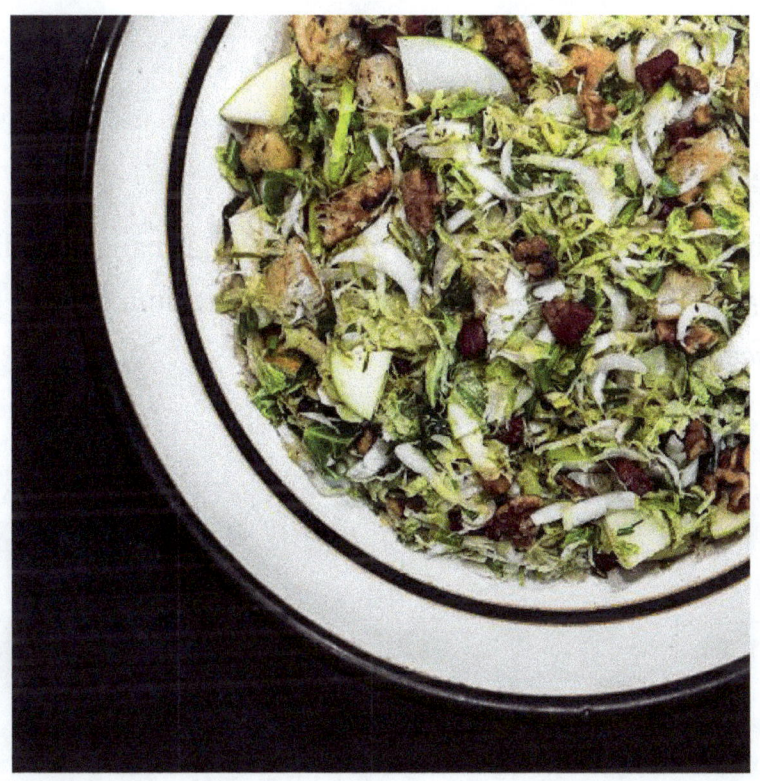

Ingredients

10 Cauliflower florets

10 pcs. Brussel Sprouts

1 bunch of endives

<u>Dressing Ingredients</u>

6 tbsp. olive oil

Sea salt, to taste

3 tbsp. white wine vinegar

1 tsp. Egg-free mayonnaise

Directions:

Marinate the vegetable with the dressing or Marinade ingredients for 15 to 30 min. Grill for 4 minutes over medium heat or until the vegetable becomes tender.

Grilled Green Bean and Microgreens in Balsamic Vinaigrette

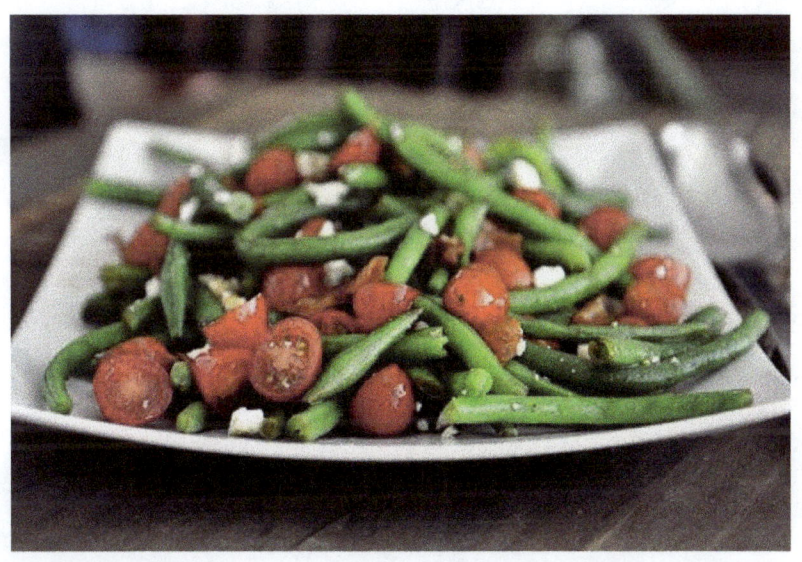

Ingredients

1 bunch of microgreens

10 Green Beans

Dressing Ingredients

6 tbsp. extra virgin olive oil

Sea salt, to taste

3 tbsp. Balsamic vinegar

1 tsp. mustard

Directions:

Marinate the vegetable with the dressing or Marinade ingredients for 15 to 30 min. Grill for 4 minutes over medium heat or until the vegetable becomes tender.

Grilled Broccolini and Turnip Greens

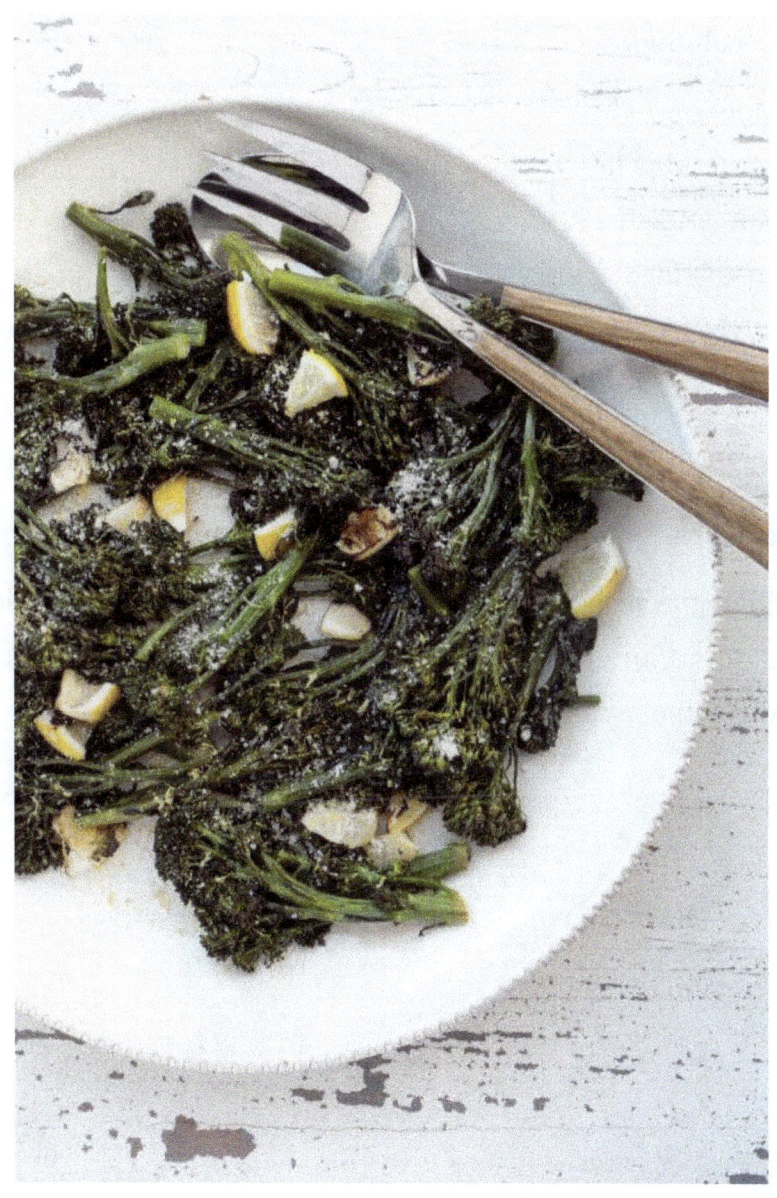

Ingredients

1 bunch of turnip greens

8 Broccolini Florets

<u>Dressing Ingredients</u>

6 tbsp. sesame oil

Sea salt, to taste

3 tbsp. distilled white vinegar

1 tsp. Egg-free mayonnaise

Directions:

Marinate the vegetable with the dressing or Marinade ingredients for 15 to 30 min. Grill for 4 minutes over medium heat or until the vegetable becomes tender.

Grilled Green Cabbage in Apple Cider Vinaigrette

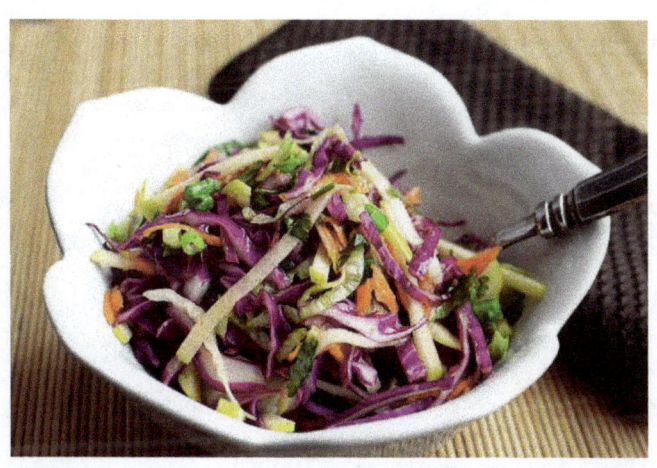

Ingredients

1 large parsnip, peeled and cut lengthwise

5 pcs. Portobello mushrooms, rinsed and drained

1 Green cabbage, cut in half

Dressing Ingredients

6 tbsp. extra virgin olive oil

Sea salt, to taste

3 tbsp. apple cider vinegar

1 tbsp. honey

1 tsp. Egg-free mayonnaise

Directions:

Marinate the vegetable with the dressing or Marinade ingredients for 15 to 30 min. Grill for 4 minutes over medium heat or until the vegetable becomes tender.

Grilled Parsnip and Rutabaga

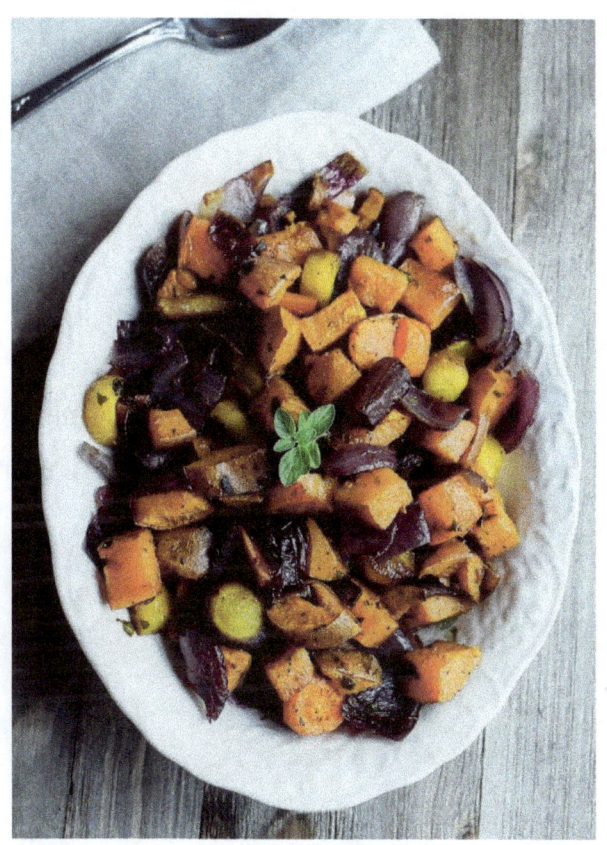

Ingredients

1 large parsnip, peeled and cut lengthwise

1 medium Rutabaga, peeled and cut in half lengthwise

2 large red onions, cut into ½ inch rings but don't separate into individual rings

Marinade ingredients:

6 tbsp. extra virgin olive oil

Sea salt, to taste

3 tbsp. distilled white vinegar

1 tsp. Dijon mustard

Directions:

Marinate the vegetable with the dressing or Marinade ingredients for 15 to 30 min. Grill for 4 minutes over medium heat or until the vegetable becomes tender.

Grilled Carrot, Turnip and Water Chestnuts with Balsamic Glaze

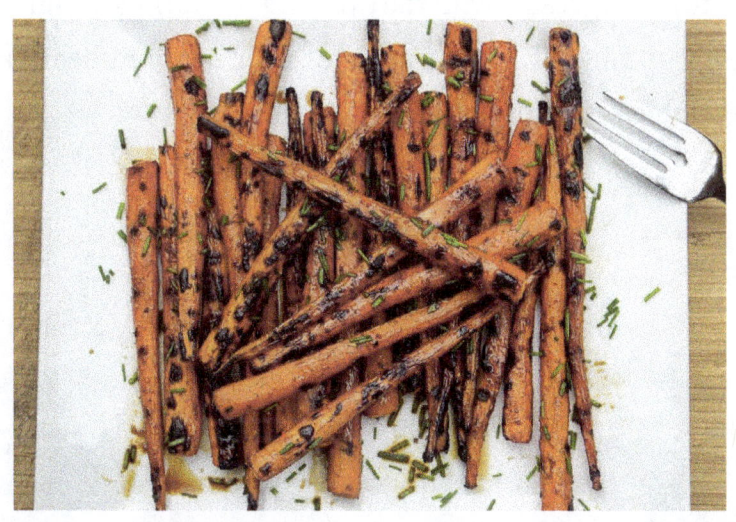

Ingredients

1 large carrots, peeled and cut lengthwise

1 large turnip, peeled and cut lengthwise

1/2 cup canned water chestnuts

2 pcs. Portobello mushrooms, rinsed and drained

<u>Dressing Ingredients</u>

6 tbsp. extra virgin olive oil

Sea salt, to taste 3 tbsp.

Balsamic vinegar 1 tsp.

Directions:

Dijon mustard

Marinate the vegetable with the dressing or Marinade ingredients for 15 to 30 min. Grill for 4 minutes over medium heat or until the vegetable becomes tender

Grilled beetroots and Green Beans

Ingredients

2 beetroots, peeled and sliced lengthwise

1 medium Pineapple, cut into

1/2 inch slices

10 Green Beans

2 large red onions, cut into ½ inch rings but don't separate into individual rings

<u>Dressing Ingredients</u>

6 tbsp. olive oil

Sea salt, to taste 3 tbsp.

white wine vinegar 1 tsp.

Directions:

English mustard Marinate the vegetable with the dressing or Marinade ingredients for 15 to 30 min. Grill for 4 minutes over medium heat or until the vegetable becomes tender.

Grilles Turnips Broccolini and Water Chestnuts with Honey Apple Cider Glaze

Ingredients

10 Broccolini Florets

1/2 cup water chestnuts

1 large turnip, peeled and cut lengthwise

<u>Dressing Ingredients</u>

6 tbsp. extra virgin olive oil

Sea salt, to taste

3 tbsp. apple cider vinegar

1 tbsp. honey

1 tsp. Egg-free mayonnaise

Directions:

Marinate the vegetable with the dressing or Marinade ingredients for 15 to 30 min. Grill for 4 minutes over medium heat or until the vegetable becomes tender.

Grilled Eggplant & Beetroot with Assorted Bell Peppers

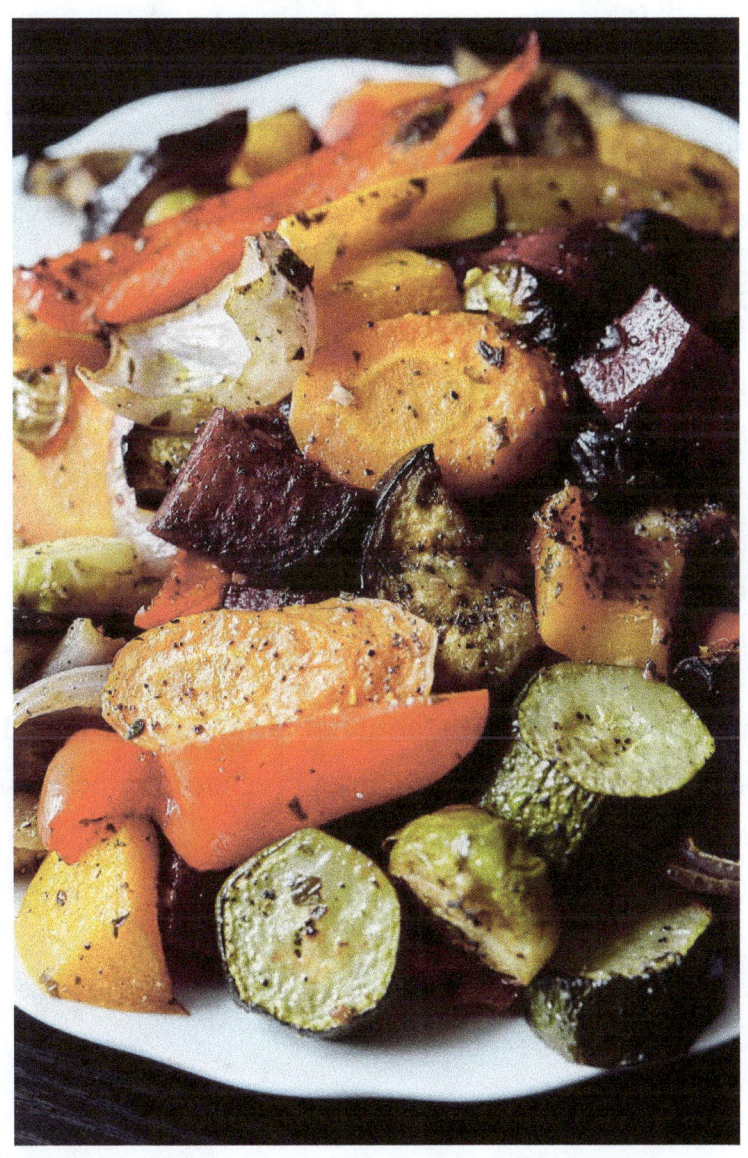

Ingredients

1 small Eggplant, cut lengthwise and cut in half

2 beetroots, peeled and sliced lengthwise

1 large turnip, peeled and cut lengthwise

1 Yellow Bell Pepper, cut in half

1 red Bell Pepper, cut in half

<u>Dressing Ingredients</u>

6 tbsp. sesame oil

Sea salt, to taste 3 tbsp.

distilled white vinegar 1 tsp.

Directions:

<u>Egg-free mayonnaise</u>

Marinate the vegetable with the dressing or Marinade ingredients for 15 to 30 min. Grill for 4 minutes over medium heat or until the vegetable becomes tender.

Grilled Water Chestnuts Zucchini and Endives

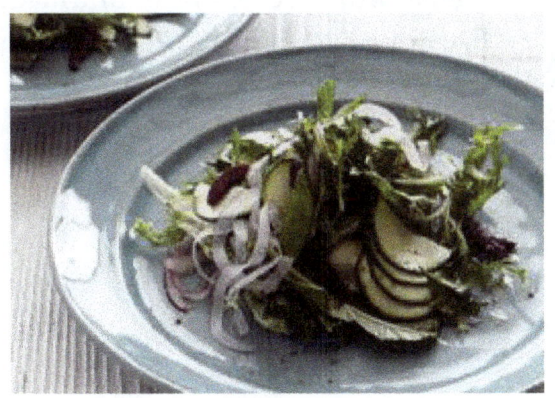

Ingredients

2 large zucchini , cut lengthwise into ½ inch slabs

1/2 cup water chestnuts

1 bunch of endives

<u>Dressing Ingredients</u>

6 tbsp. sesame oil

Sea salt, to taste 3 tbsp.

distilled white vinegar 1 tsp.

Directions:

<u>Egg-free mayonnaise</u>

Marinate the vegetable with the dressing or Marinade ingredients for 15 to 30 min. Grill for 4 minutes over medium heat or until the vegetable becomes tender.

Grilled Collard Greens Portobello and Asparagus

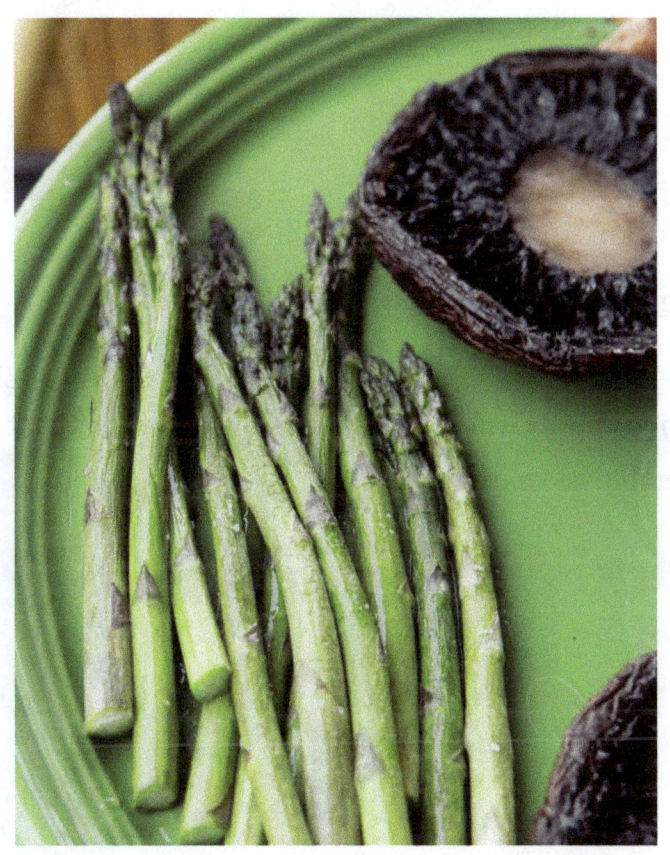

Ingredients

3 pcs. Portobello, rinsed and drained

1 medium Rutabaga, peeled and cut in half lengthwise

1 bunch of collard greens

6 pcs. Asparagus

Dressing Ingredients

6 tbsp. sesame oil

Sea salt, to taste 3 tbsp.

distilled white vinegar 1 tsp.

Directions:

Egg-free mayonnaise

Marinate the vegetable with the dressing or marinade ingredients for 15 to 30 min. Grill for 4 minutes over medium heat or until the vegetable becomes tender.

Grilled Ruttabaga and Swiss Chard

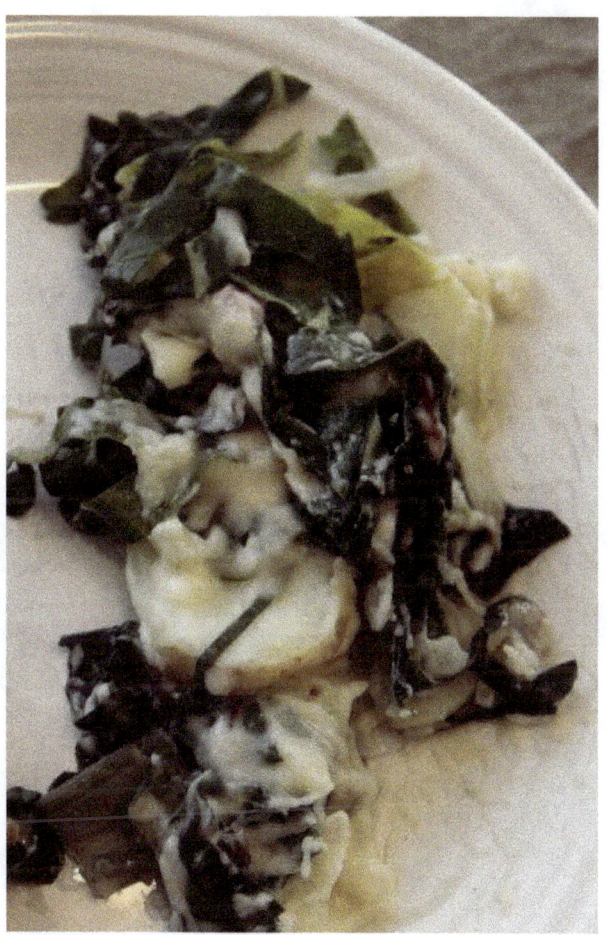

Ingredients

1 medium Rutabaga, peeled and cut in half lengthwise

2 large red onions, cut into ½ inch rings but don't separate into individual rings

1 bunch of swiss chard

Marinade ingredients:

6 tbsp. extra virgin olive oil

Sea salt, to taste

3 tbsp. distilled white vinegar

1 tsp. Dijon mustard

Directions:

Marinate the vegetable with the dressing or marinade ingredients for 15 to 30 min. Grill for 4 minutes over medium heat or until the vegetable becomes tender.

Grilled Green Beans and Eggplants

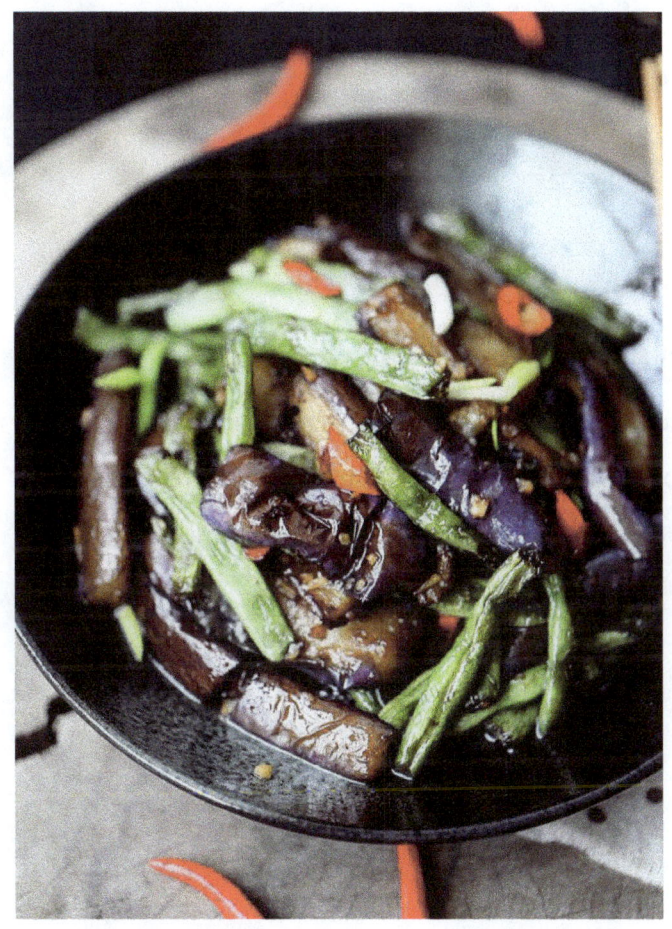

Ingredients

2 beetroots, peeled and sliced lengthwise

2 large Zucchinis, cut lengthwise and cut in half

10 Green Beans

Dressing Ingredients

6 tbsp. extra virgin olive oil

Sea salt, to taste 3 tbsp.

Balsamic vinegar 1 tsp.

Directions:

Dijon mustard

Marinate the vegetable with the dressing or Marinade ingredients for 15 to 30 min. Grill for 4 minutes over medium heat or until the vegetable becomes tender.

Grilled Collard Greens and Brussel Sprouts

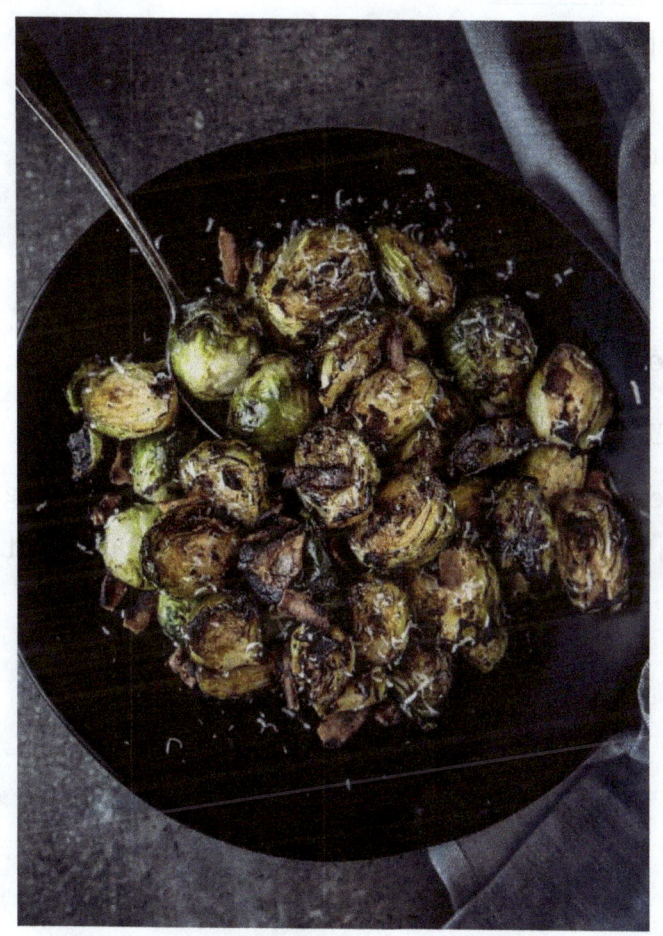

Ingredients

1 bunch of collard greens

10 pcs. Brussel Sprouts

10 Broccolini Florets

1 bunch of swiss chard

Dressing Ingredients

6 tbsp. olive oil

Sea salt, to taste 3 tbsp.

white wine vinegar 1 tsp.

Directions:

English mustard

Marinate the vegetable with the dressing or Marinade ingredients for 15 to 30 min. Grill for 4 minutes over medium heat or until the vegetable becomes tender.

Grilled Swiss Chard and Asparagus

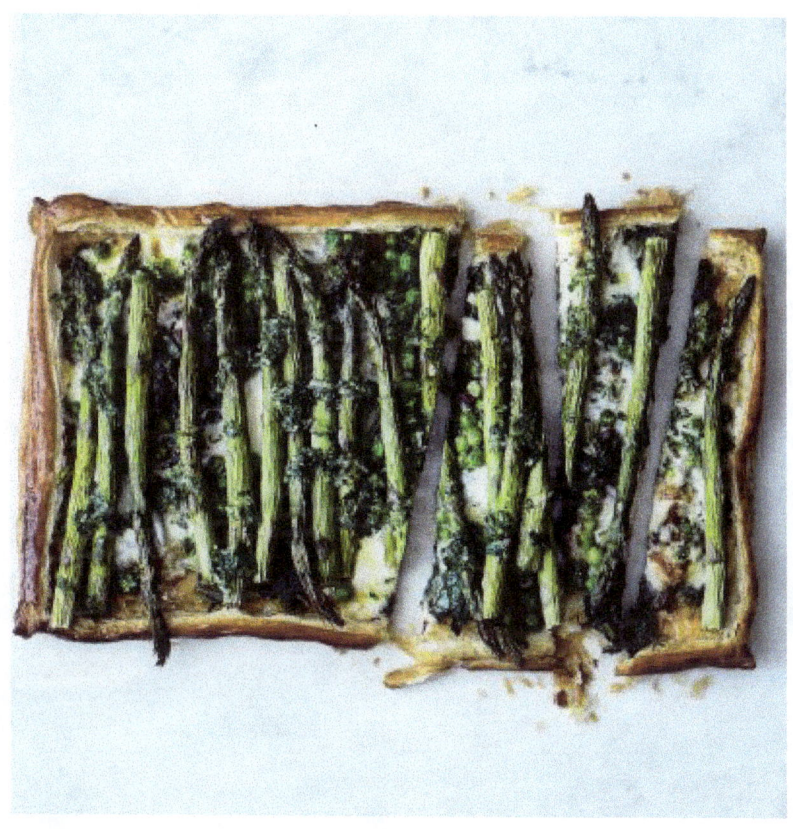

Ingredients

1 medium Rutabaga, peeled and cut in half lengthwise

2 large red onions, cut into ½ inch rings but don't separate into individual rings

1 bunch of swiss chard

10 pcs. Asparagus

Dressing Ingredients

6 tbsp. extra virgin olive oil

Sea salt, to taste 3 tbsp.

apple cider vinegar 1 tbsp.

honey 1 tsp.

Directions:

Egg-free mayonnaise

Marinate the vegetable with the dressing or Marinade ingredients for 15 to 30 min. Grill for 4 minutes over medium heat or until the vegetable becomes tender.

Grilled Endives and Edamame Beans

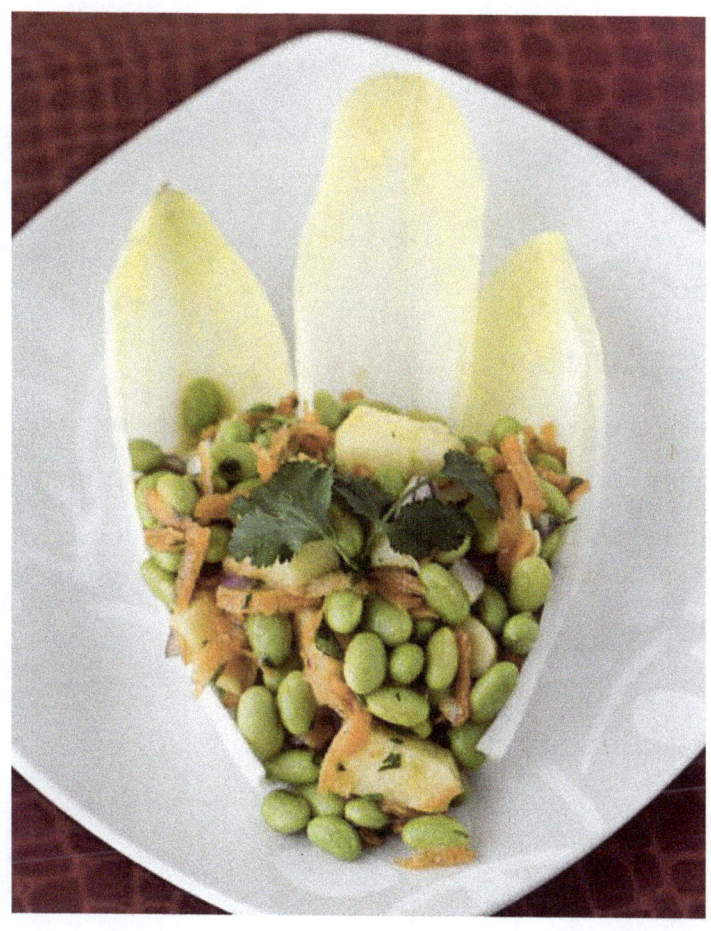

Ingredients

10 Edamame Beans

2 beetroots, peeled and sliced lengthwise

1 bunch of endives

Dressing Ingredients

6 tbsp. olive oil

Sea salt, to taste 3 tbsp.

white wine vinegar 1 tsp.

Directions:

Egg-free mayonnaise

Marinate the vegetable with the dressing or Marinade ingredients for 15 to 30 min. Grill for 4 minutes over medium heat or until the vegetable becomes tender.

Grilled Water Chestnuts and Cabbage

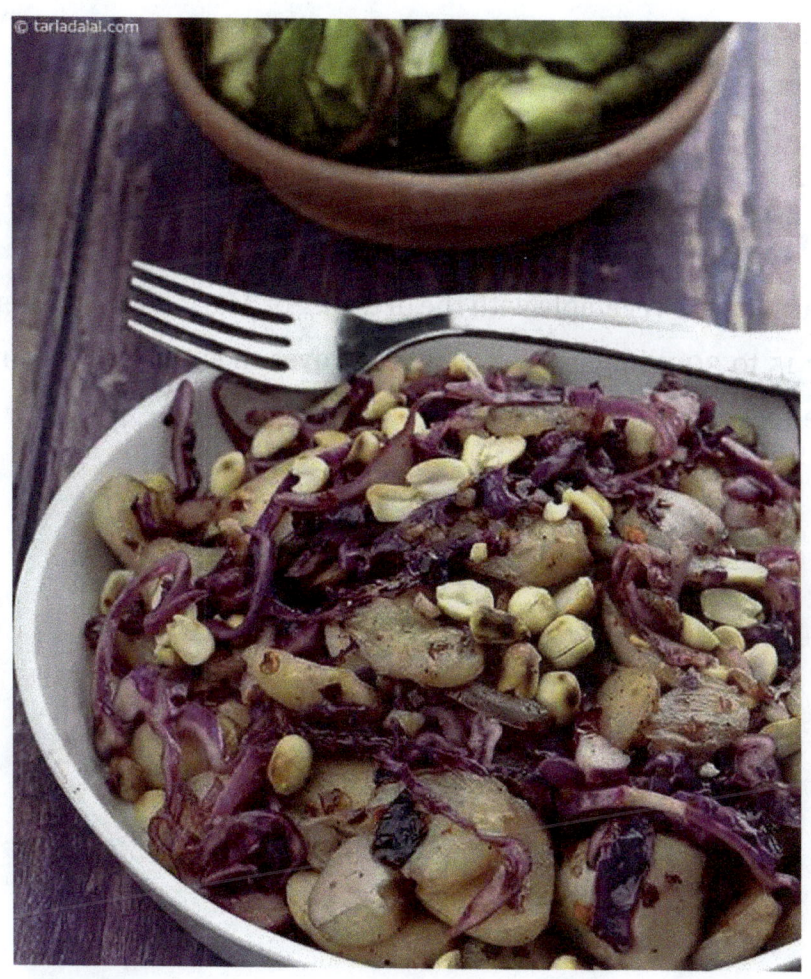

Ingredients

1 Green cabbage

1/2 cup water chestnuts

2 large red onions, cut into ½ inch rings but don't separate into

individual rings

2 tbsp. extra virgin olive oil

2 tbsp. ranch dressing mix

Directions:

Marinate the vegetable with the dressing or Marinade ingredients for 15 to 30 min. Grill for 4 minutes over medium heat or until the vegetable becomes tender.

Grilled Okra and Waterchestnuts

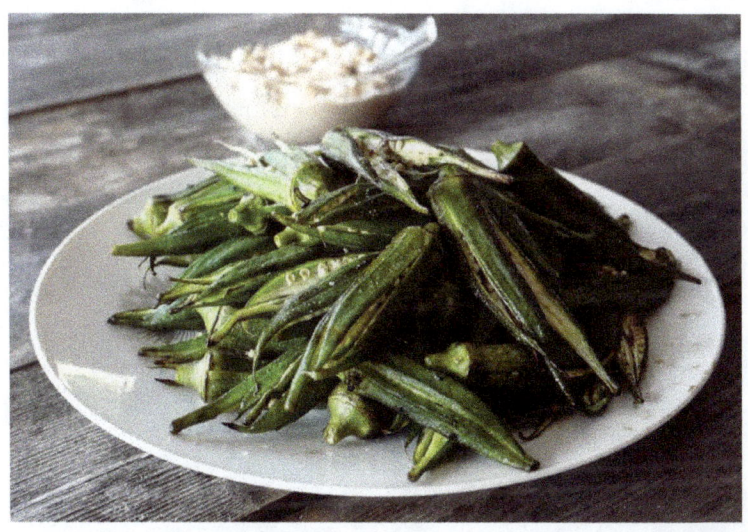

Ingredients

1 red cabbage

1/2 cup water chestnuts

5 pcs. Okra

3 pcs. Asparagus Corns, cut lengthwise

2 pcs. Portobello mushrooms, rinsed and drained Marinade ingredients:

6 tbsp. extra virgin olive oil

Sea salt, to taste 3 tbsp.

distilled white vinegar 1 tsp.

Directions:

<u>Dijon mustard</u>

Marinate the vegetable with the dressing or Marinade ingredients for 15 to 30 min. Grill for 4 minutes over medium heat or until the vegetable becomes tender.

Grilled Turnip Greens and Broccolini

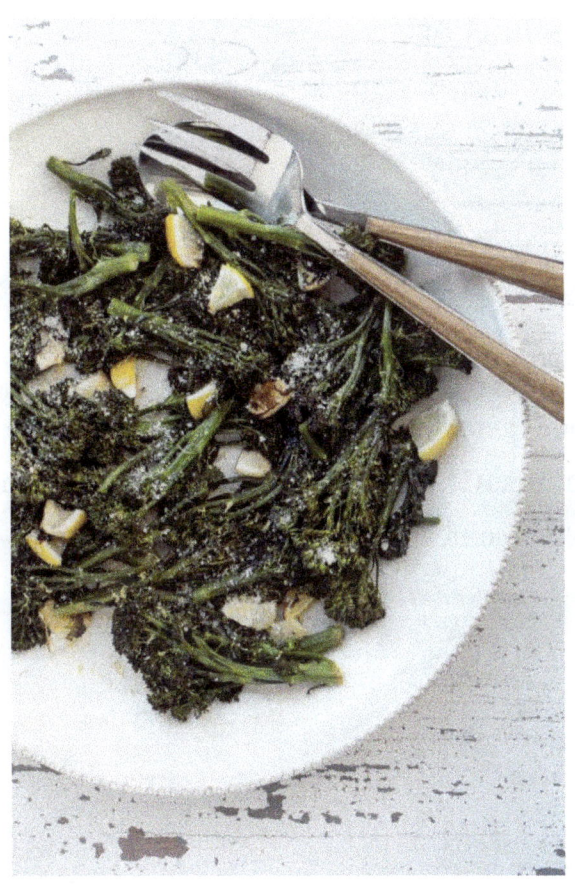

Ingredients

1 bunch of turnip greens

10 pcs. Brussel Sprouts

10 Broccolini Florets

10 pcs. Asparagus

Dressing Ingredients

6 tbsp. sesame oil

Sea salt, to taste 3 tbsp.

distilled white vinegar 1 tsp.

Directions:

Egg-free mayonnaise

Marinate the vegetable with the dressing or Marinade ingredients for 15 to 30 min. Grill for 4 minutes over medium heat or until the vegetable becomes tender.

Grilled Parsnip and Microgreens

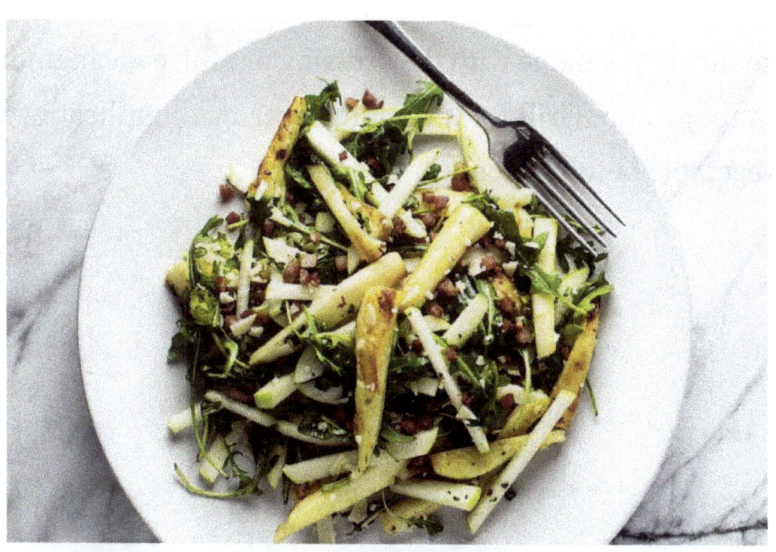

Ingredients

1 large Parsnip, cut lengthwise

1 bunch of microgreens

2 large red onions, cut into ½ inch rings but don't separate into individual rings

Dressing Ingredients

6 tbsp. olive oil

Sea salt, to taste 3 tbsp.

white wine vinegar 1 tsp.

Directions:

Egg-free mayonnaise

Marinate the vegetable with the dressing or Marinade ingredients for 15 to 30 min. Grill for 4 minutes over medium heat or until the vegetable becomes tender.

Grilled Carrot, Parsnip and Endives

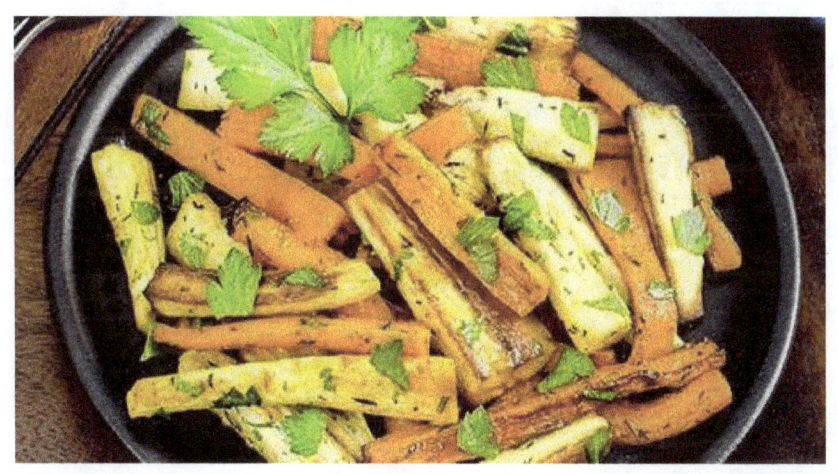

Ingredients

1 large Carrot, cut lengthwise

1 large Parsnip, cut lengthwise

1 bunch of endives

10 pcs. Asparagus

10 Green Beans

Dressing Ingredients

6 tbsp. olive oil

Sea salt, to taste 3 tbsp.

white wine vinegar 1 tsp.

Directions:

English mustard

Marinate the vegetable with the dressing or Marinade ingredients for 15 to 30 min. Grill for 4 minutes over medium heat or until the vegetable becomes tender.

Grilled Cauliflower and Baby Corn

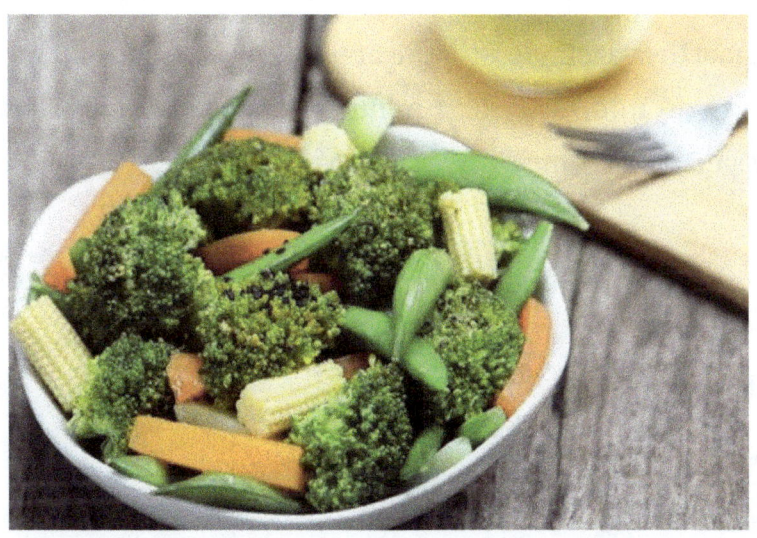

Ingredients

10 Cauliflower florets

½ cup canned baby corn

10 pcs. Brussel Sprouts

Dressing Ingredients

6 tbsp. extra virgin olive oil

Sea salt, to taste 3 tbsp.

apple cider vinegar 1 tbsp.

honey 1 tsp.

Directions:

Egg-free mayonnaise

Marinate the vegetable with the dressing or Marinade ingredients for 15 to 30 min. Grill for 4 minutes over medium heat or until the vegetable becomes tender.

Grilled Baby Carrots and Beetroots

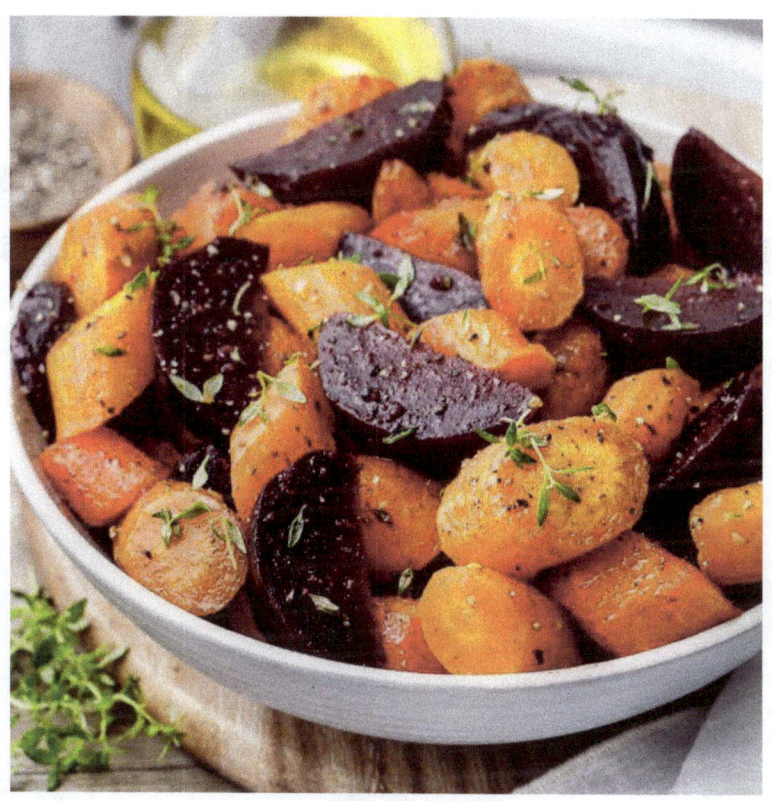

Ingredients

5 pcs. baby carrots

2 large Eggplants, cut lengthwise and cut in half

2 beetroots, peeled and sliced lengthwise

Dressing Ingredients

6 tbsp. sesame oil

Sea salt, to taste

3 tbsp. distilled white vinegar

1 tsp. Egg-free mayonnaise

Directions:

Marinate the vegetable with the dressing or Marinade ingredients for 15 to 30 min. Grill for 4 minutes over medium heat or until the vegetable becomes tender.

Grilled Microgreens and Beetroots

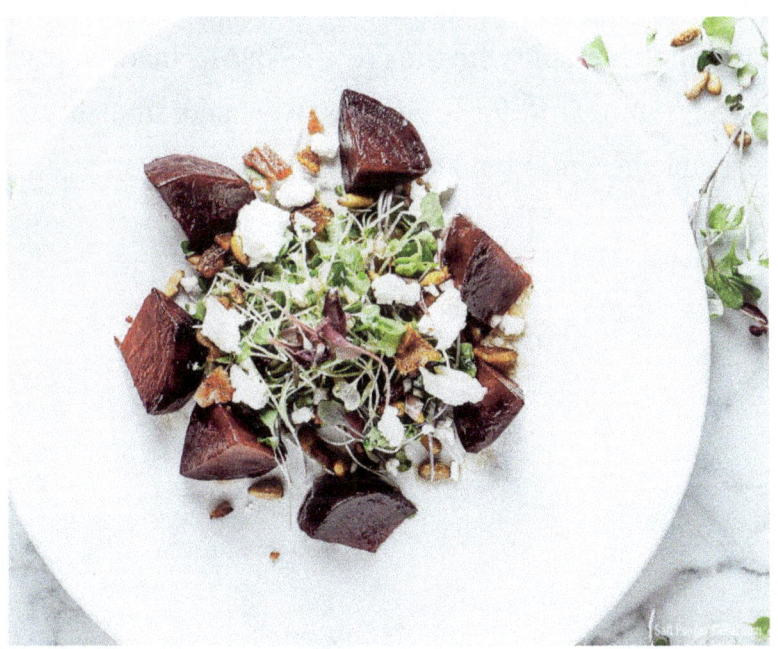

Ingredients

1 bunch of microgreens

2 beetroots, peeled and sliced lengthwise Corns, cut lengthwise

Dressing Ingredients

6 tbsp. extra virgin olive oil

Sea salt, to taste 3 tbsp.

Balsamic vinegar 1 tsp.

Directions:

Dijon mustard

Marinate the vegetable with the dressing or Marinade ingredients for 15 to 30 min. Grill for 4 minutes over medium heat or until the vegetable becomes tender.

Grilled Rutabaga Pineapple and Artichoke Hearts

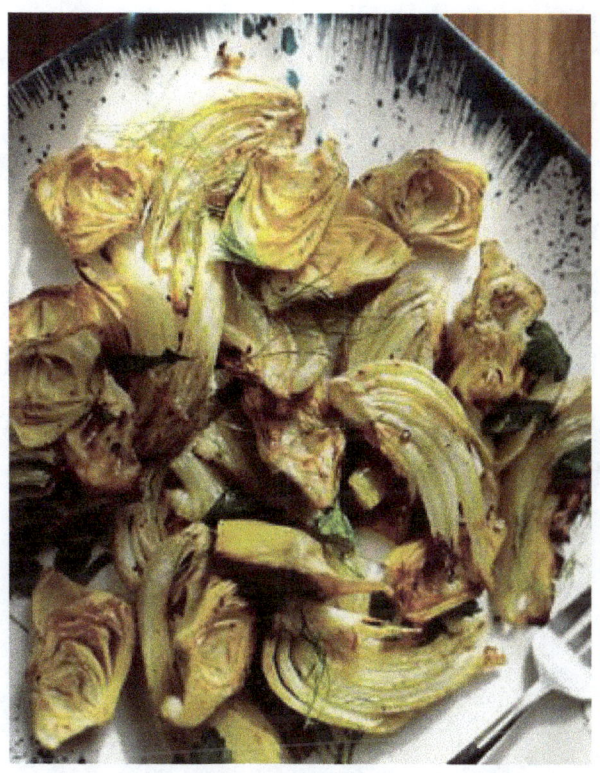

Ingredients

1 medium Pineapple, cut into 1/2 inch slices

1 medium Rutabaga, peeled and cut in half lengthwise

1 cup canned artichoke hearts

Marinade ingredients:

6 tbsp. extra virgin olive oil

Sea salt, to taste 3 tbsp.

distilled white vinegar 1 tsp.

Directions:

Dijon mustard

Marinate the vegetable with the dressing or Marinade ingredients for 15 to 30 min. Grill for 4 minutes over medium heat or until the vegetable becomes tender.

Simple Grilled Water Chestnuts and Cauliflower Florets

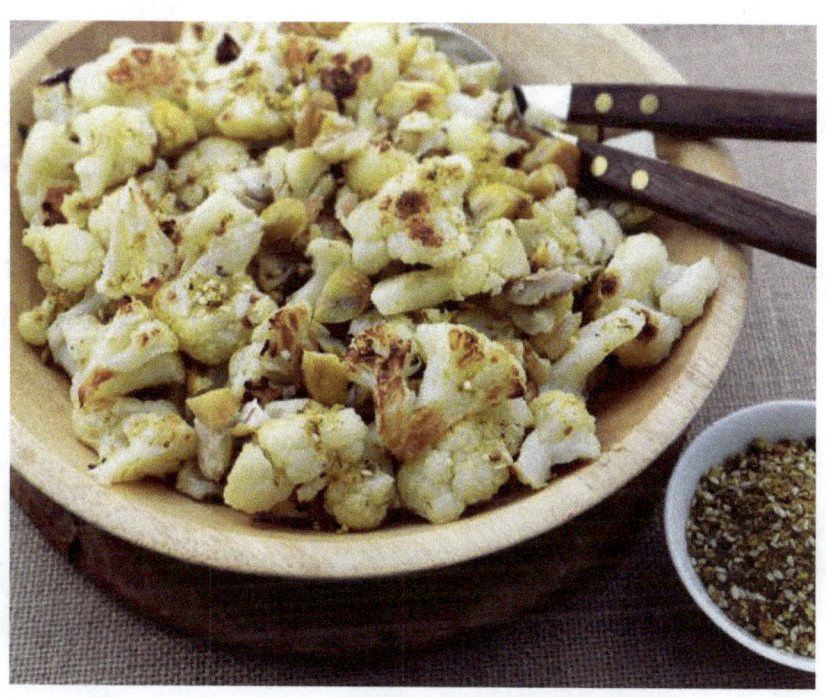

Ingredients

1/2 cup canned water chestnuts

10 Cauliflower florets

10 pcs. Brussel Sprouts

Dressing Ingredients

6 tbsp. extra virgin olive oil

Sea salt, to taste 3 tbsp.

apple cider vinegar 1 tbsp.

honey 1 tsp.

Directions:

<u>Egg-free mayonnaise</u>

Marinate the vegetable with the dressing or Marinade ingredients for 15 to 30 min. Grill for 4 minutes over medium heat or until the vegetable becomes tender.

Grilled Baby Corn, Water Chestnuts and Eggplant

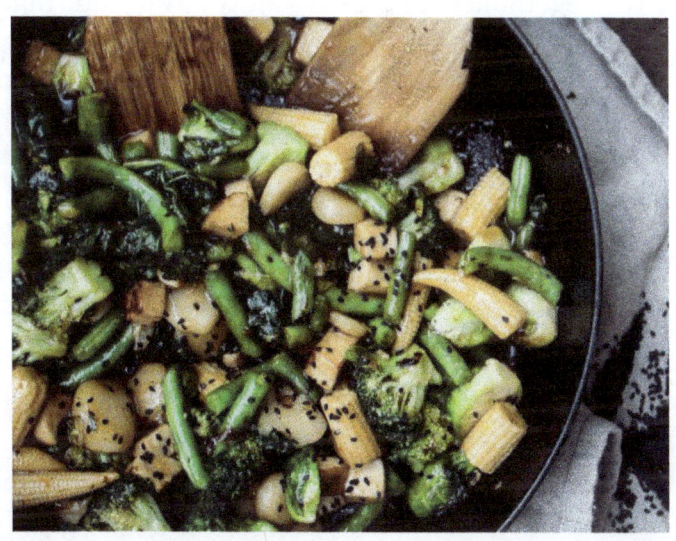

Ingredients

½ cup canned baby corn

1/2 cup canned water chestnuts

2 large Eggplants, cut lengthwise and cut in half

Dressing Ingredients

6 tbsp. olive oil

Sea salt, to taste 3 tbsp.

white wine vinegar 1 tsp.

Directions:

<u>Egg-free mayonnaise</u>

Marinate the vegetable with the dressing or Marinade ingredients for 15 to 30 min. Grill for 4 minutes over medium heat or until the vegetable becomes tender.

Grilled Broccolini Beetroots and Portobello Mushroom

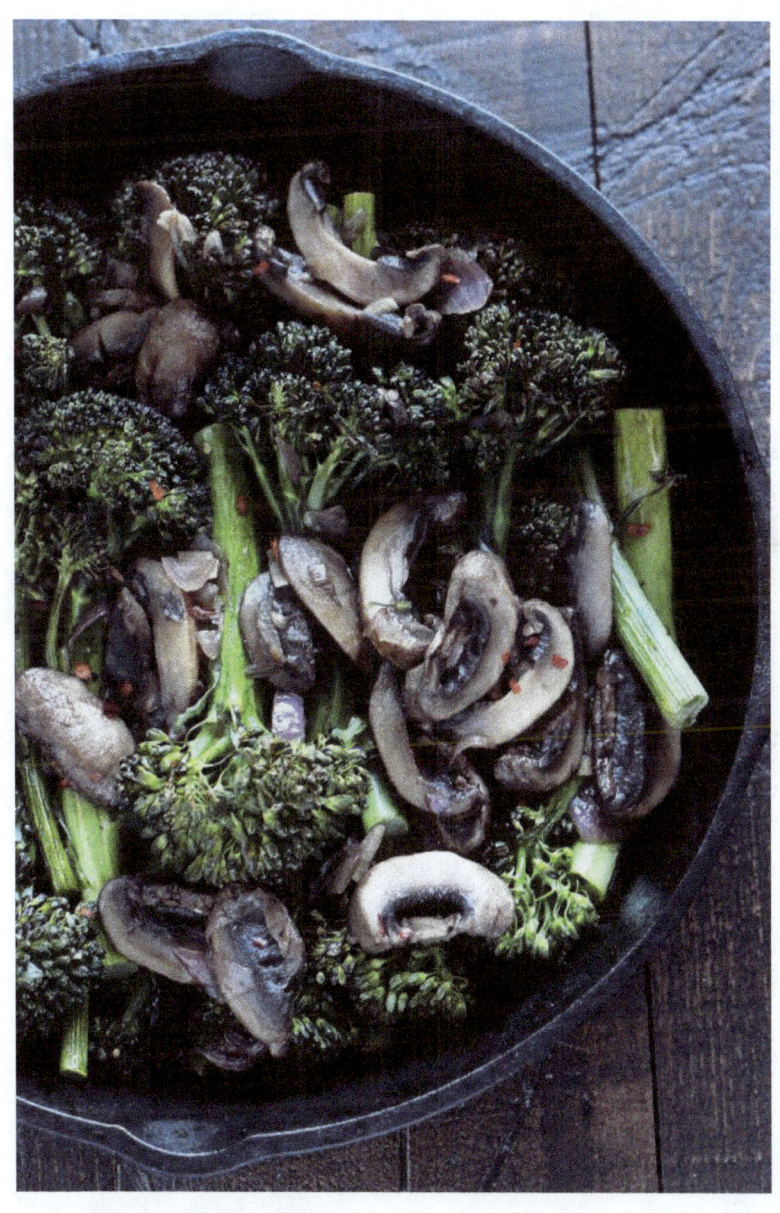

Ingredients

10 Broccolini Florets

2 beetroots, peeled and sliced lengthwise Corns, cut lengthwise

5 pcs. Portobello mushrooms, rinsed and drained

<u>Dressing Ingredients</u>

6 tbsp. sesame oil

Sea salt, to taste 3 tbsp.

distilled white vinegar 1 tsp.

Directions:

<u>Egg-free mayonnaise</u>

Marinate the vegetable with the dressing or Marinade ingredients for 15 to 30 min. Grill for 4 minutes over medium heat or until the vegetable becomes tender.

Grilled Baby Carrots and Baby Carrots

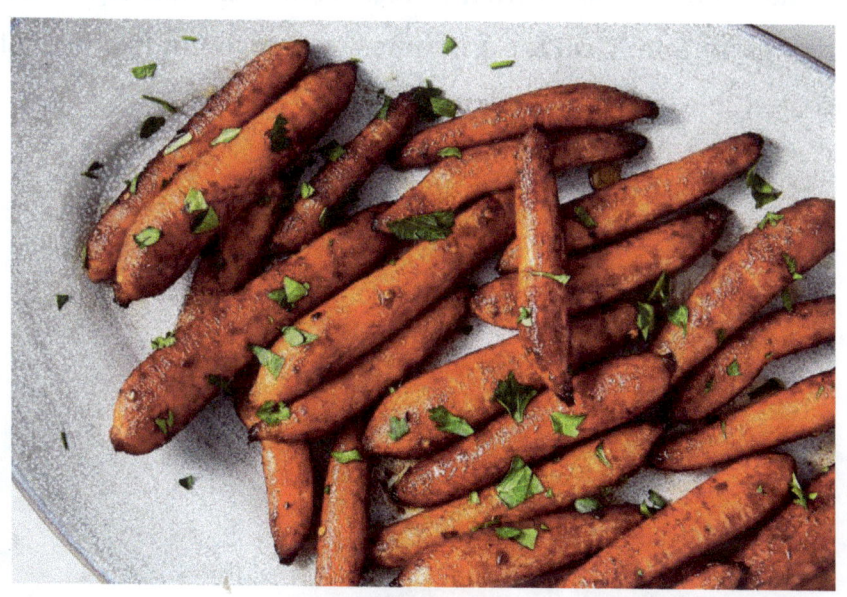

Ingredients

10 pcs. Baby Carrots

2 beetroots, peeled and sliced lengthwise

Dressing Ingredients

6 tbsp. olive oil

Sea salt, to taste

3 tbsp. white wine vinegar

1 tsp. Egg-free mayonnaise

Directions:

Marinate the vegetable with the dressing or Marinade ingredients for 15 to 30 min. Grill for 4 minutes over medium heat or until the vegetable becomes tender.

Grilled Turnip Greens

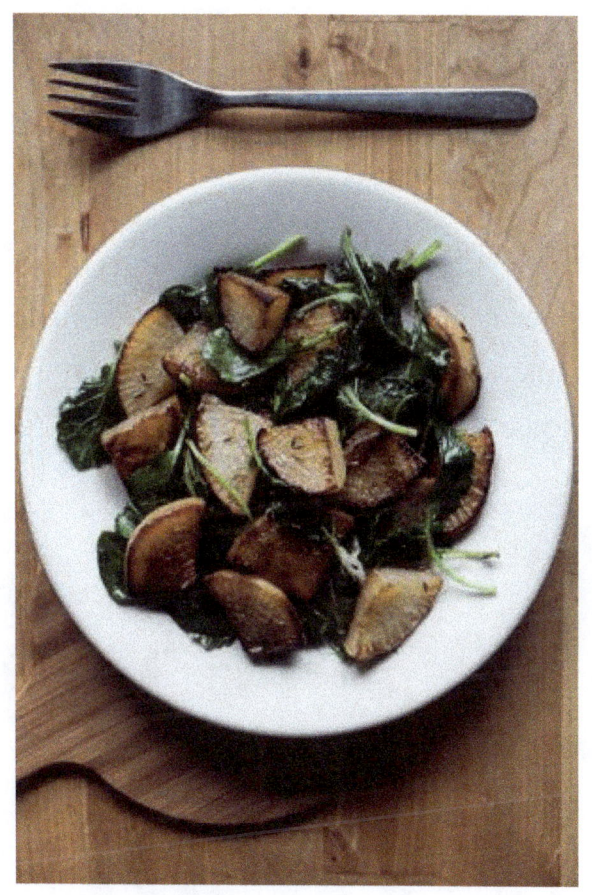

Ingredients

1 bunch of turnip greens

Dressing Ingredients

6 tbsp. olive oil

Sea salt, to taste 3 tbsp.

white wine vinegar 1 tsp.

Directions:

<u>Egg-free mayonnaise</u>

Marinate the vegetable with the dressing or Marinade ingredients for 15 to 30 min. Grill for 4 minutes over medium heat or until the vegetable becomes tender.

Grilled Broccolini Florets and Summer Squash

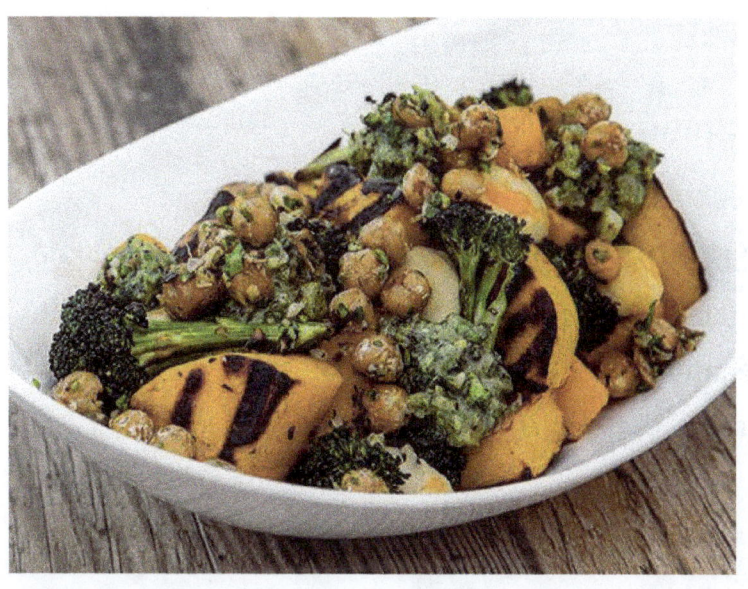

Ingredients

10 Broccolini Florets

10 pcs. Brussel Sprouts

10 pcs. Asparagus

1 summer squash, peeled and sliced lengthwise

4 large Tomatoes, sliced thick

Dressing Ingredients:

6 tbsp. extra virgin olive oil

1 tsp. onion powder

Sea salt, to taste 3 tbsp.

distilled white vinegar 1 tsp.

Directions:

<u>Dijon mustard</u>

Combine all of the dressing ingredients thoroughly. Preheat your grill to low heat and grease the grates. Layer the vegetables grill for 12 minutes per side, until tender flipping once. Brush with the marinade/ dressing ingredients

Grilled Winter Squash and Eggplant

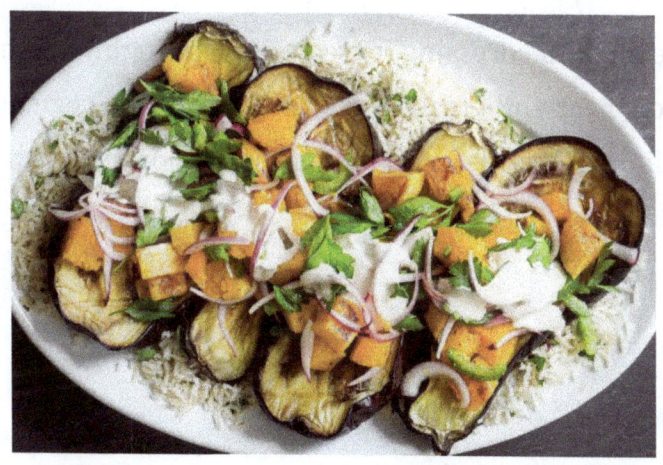

Ingredients

1 lb eggplant, sliced lengthwise into shorter sticks

1 winter squash, peeled and sliced lengthwise

1 large red onion, cut into 1/2 inch thick rounds

1/3 cup Italian parsley or basil, finely chopped

Dressing Ingredients:

6 tbsp. extra virgin olive oil

1 tsp. onion powder

Sea salt, to taste 3 tbsp.

distilled white vinegar 1 tsp.

Directions:

<u>Dijon mustard</u>

Combine all of the dressing ingredients thoroughly. Preheat your grill to low heat and grease the grates. Layer the vegetables grill for 12 minutes per side, until tender flipping once. Brush with the marinade/ dressing ingredients

Grilled Zucchini and Green Bell Peppers

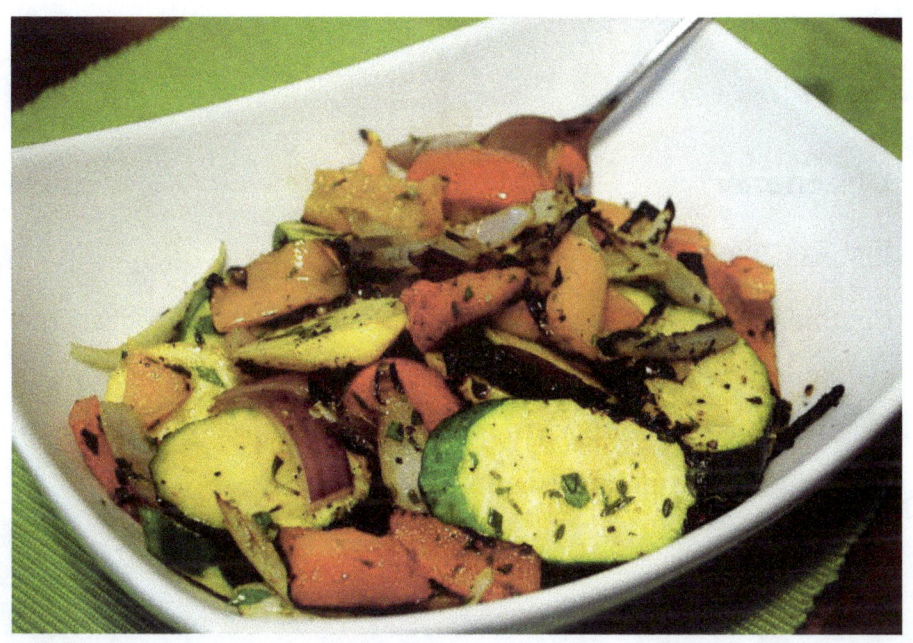

Ingredients

1 lb zucchini, sliced lengthwise into shorter sticks

1 lb green bell peppers, sliced into wide strips

1 large red onion, cut into

1/2 inch thick rounds

1/3 cup Italian parsley or basil, finely chopped

Dressing Ingredients

6 tbsp. extra virgin olive oil

Sea salt, to taste 3 tbsp.

apple cider vinegar 1 tbsp.

honey 1 tsp.

Directions:

<u>Egg-free mayonnaise</u>

Combine all of the dressing ingredients thoroughly. Preheat your grill to low heat and grease the grates. Layer the vegetables grill for 12 minutes per side, until tender flipping once. Brush with the marinade/ dressing ingredients

Grilled Zucchini & Butternut Squash

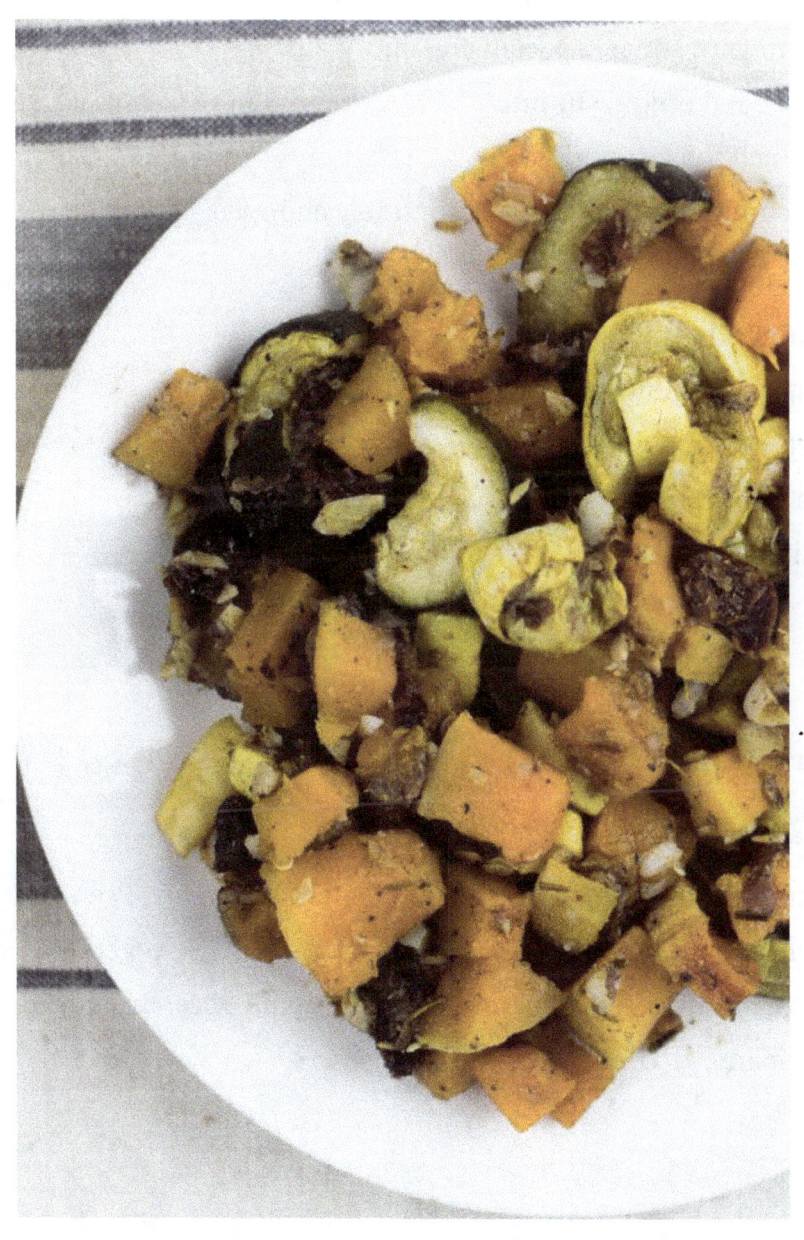

Ingredients

1 lb zucchini, sliced lengthwise into shorter sticks

1 butternut squash, peeled and sliced len

1 large red onion, cut into

1/2 inch thick rounds

1/3 cup Italian parsley or basil, finely chopped

Dressing Ingredients

6 tbsp. olive oil

1 tsp. garlic powder

1 tsp. onion powder

Sea salt, to taste 3 tbsp.

white wine vinegar 1 tsp.

Directions:

English mustard

Combine all of the dressing ingredients thoroughly. Preheat your grill to low heat and grease the grates. Layer the vegetables grill for 12 minutes per side, until tender flipping once. Brush with the marinade/ dressing ingredients

Grilled Baby Corn Zucchini and Beetroots

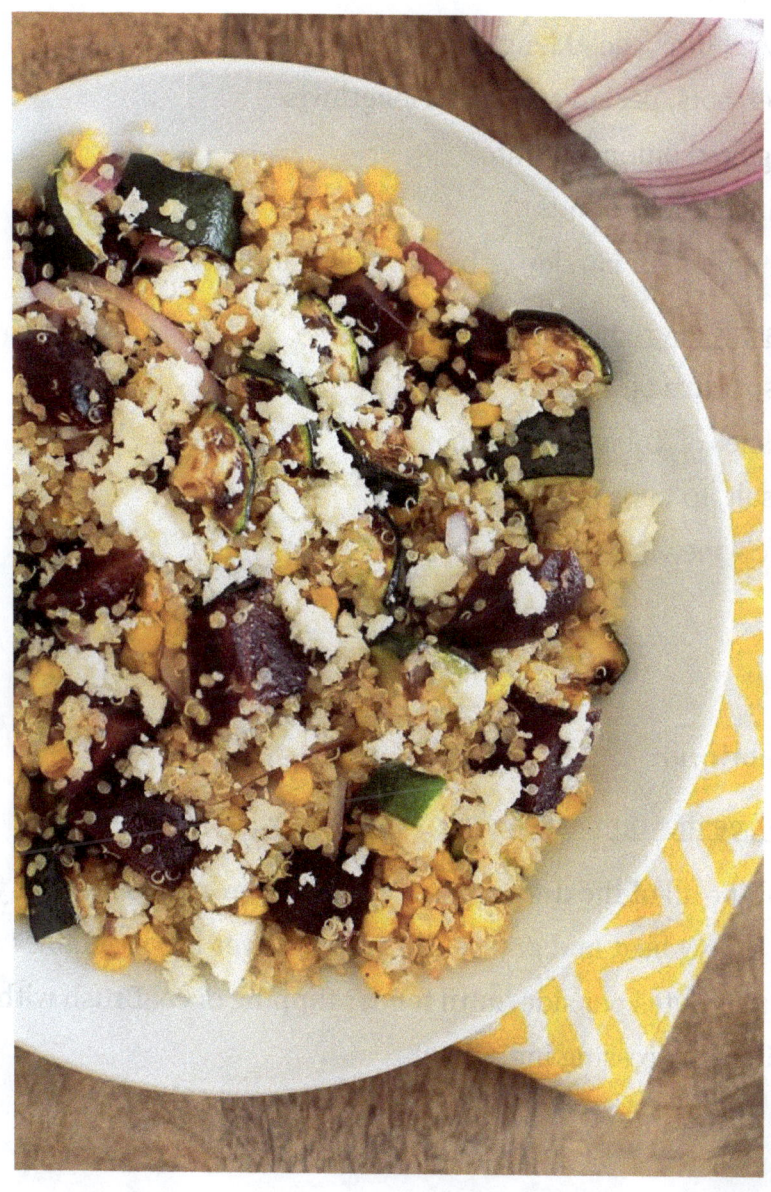

Ingredients

½ cup baby corn

1 lb zucchini, sliced lengthwise into shorter sticks

2 beetroots, peeled and sliced lengthwise

1 large red onion, cut into

1/2 inch thick rounds

1/3 cup Italian parsley or basil, finely chopped

<u>Dressing Ingredients</u>

6 tbsp. olive oil

3 dashes of Tabasco hot sauce

Sea salt, to taste 3 tbsp.

white wine vinegar 1 tsp.

Directions:

<u>Egg-free mayonnaise</u>

Combine all of the dressing ingredients thoroughly. Preheat your grill to low heat and grease the grates. Layer the vegetables grill for 12 minutes per side, until tender flipping once. Brush with the marinade/ dressing ingredients

Grilled Summer Squash and Carrots

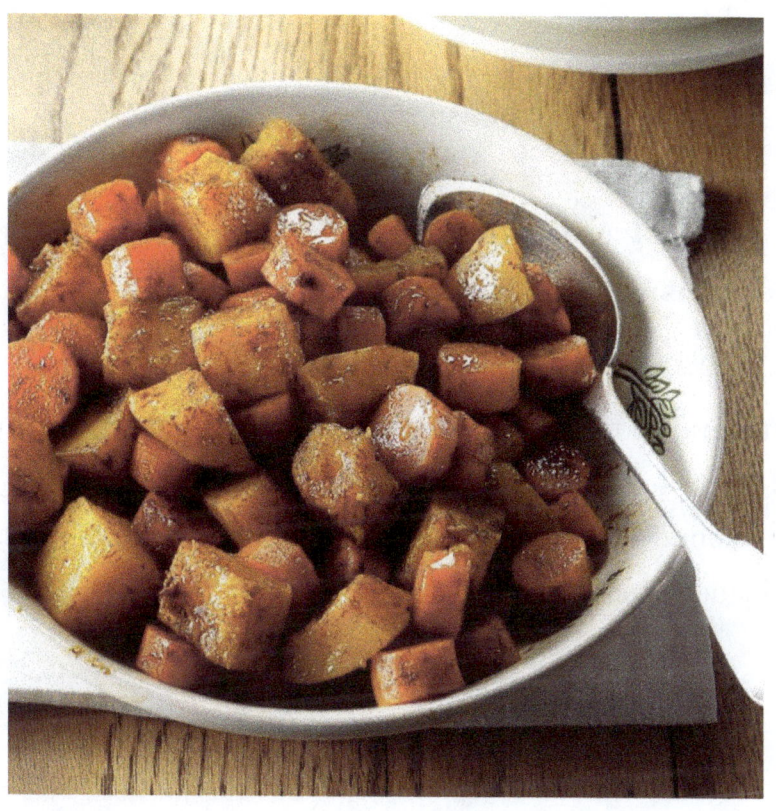

Ingredients

1 summer squash, peeled and sliced lengthwise

1 baby carrots, rinsed

1 large red onion, cut into

1/2 inch thick rounds

1/3 cup Italian parsley or basil, finely chopped

Dressing Ingredients

6 tbsp. extra virgin olive oil

Sea salt, to taste 3 tbsp.

Balsamic vinegar 1 tsp.

Directions:

Dijon mustard

Combine all of the dressing ingredients thoroughly. Preheat your grill to low heat and grease the grates. Layer the vegetables grill for 12 minutes per side, until tender flipping once. Brush with the marinade/ dressing ingredients

Grilled Edamame Beans and Zucchini

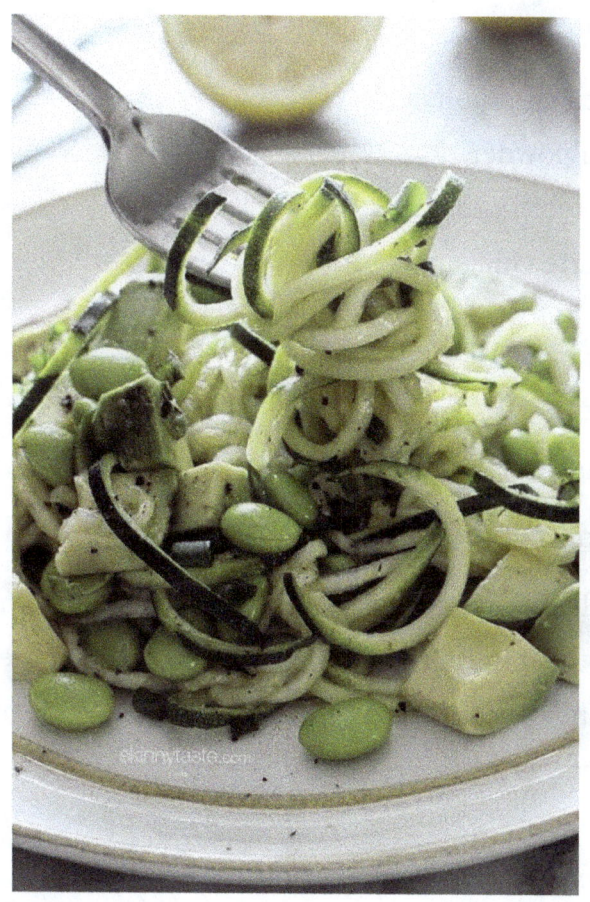

Ingredients

20 pcs. Edamame Beans

1 lb zucchini, sliced lengthwise into shorter sticks

1 lb green bell peppers, sliced into wide strips

1 large red onion, cut into

1/2 inch thick rounds

1/3 cup Italian parsley or basil, finely chopped

Dressing Ingredients:

6 tbsp. extra virgin olive oil

1 tsp. onion powder

Sea salt, to taste 3 tbsp.

distilled white vinegar 1 tsp.

Directions:

Dijon mustard

Combine all of the dressing ingredients thoroughly. Preheat your grill to low heat and grease the grates. Layer the vegetables grill for 12 minutes per side, until tender flipping once. Brush with the marinade/ dressing ingredients

Grilled Okra and Mustard Greens

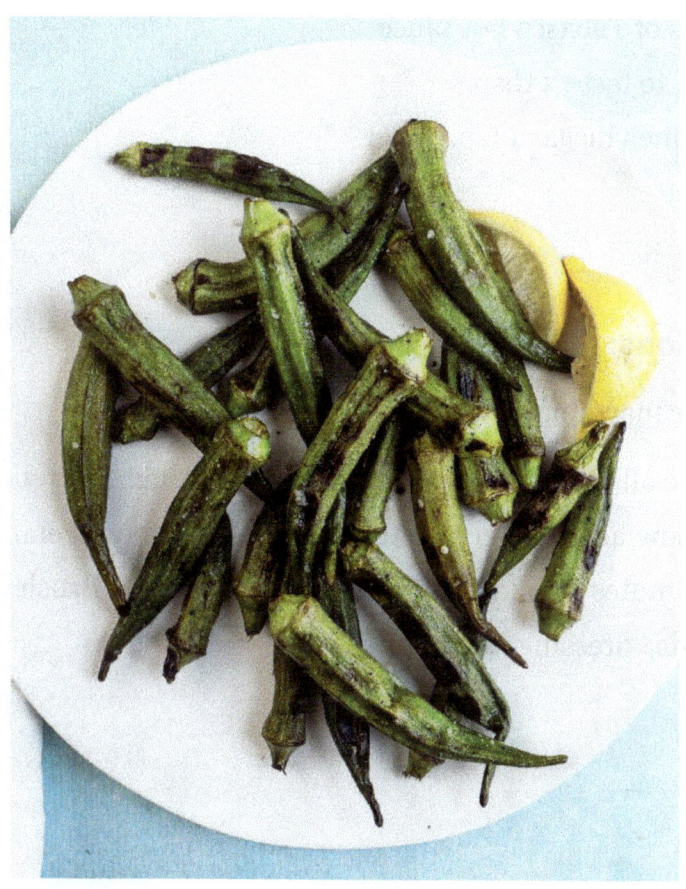

Ingredients

10 pcs. Okra

1 bunch of mustard greens

10 pcs. Brussel Sprouts

1 large red onion, cut into 1/2 inch thick rounds

1/3 cup Italian parsley or basil, finely chopped

Dressing Ingredients

6 tbsp. olive oil

3 dashes of Tabasco hot sauce

Sea salt, to taste 3 tbsp.

white wine vinegar 1 tsp.

Directions:

Egg-free mayonnaise

Combine all of the dressing ingredients thoroughly. Preheat your grill to low heat and grease the grates. Layer the vegetables grill for 12 minutes per side, until tender flipping once. Brush with the marinade/ dressing ingredients

Grilled Beetroots & Kale

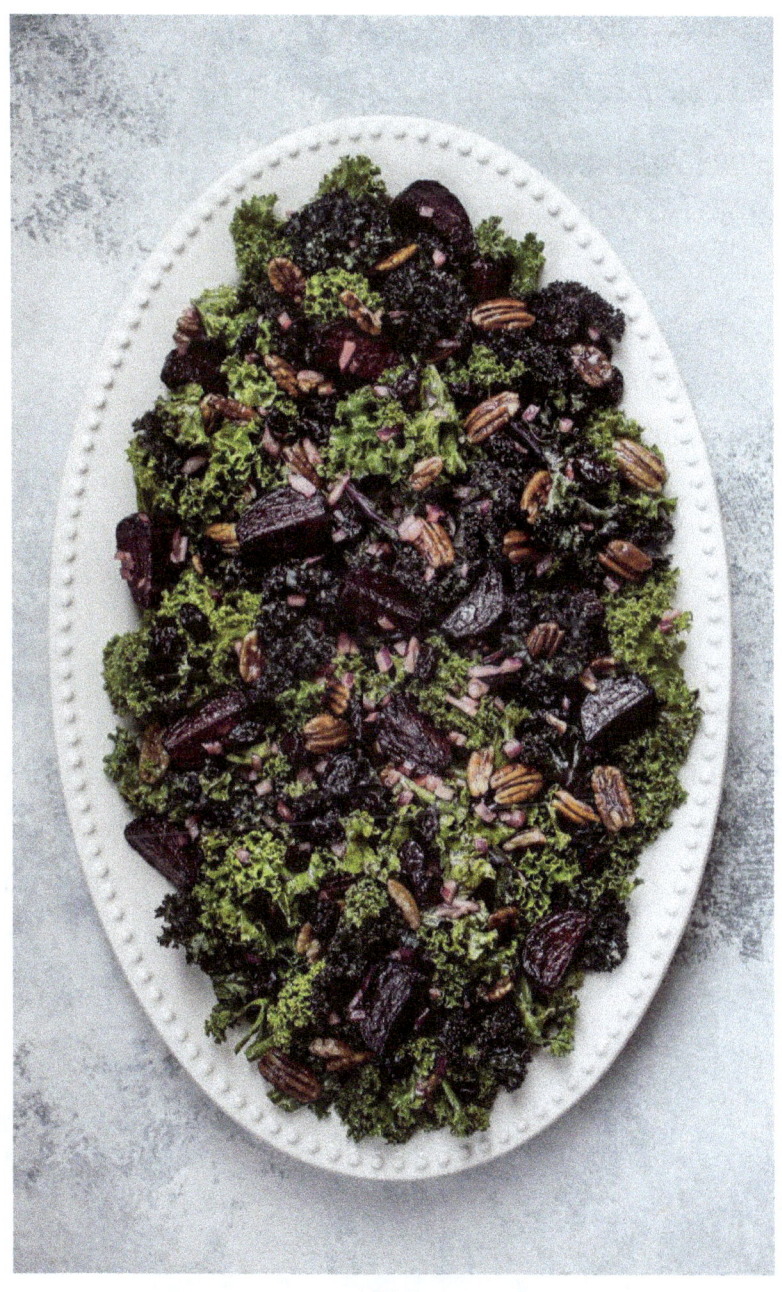

Ingredients

1 bunch of Kale

2 beetroots, peeled and sliced lengthwise

1/3 cup Italian parsley or basil, finely chopped

<u>Dressing Ingredients</u>

6 tbsp. extra virgin olive oil

Sea salt, to taste 1 tsp.

onion powder 1/2 tsp.

Herbs de Provence 3 tbsp.

white vinegar 1 tsp.

Directions:

<u>Dijon mustard</u>

Combine all of the dressing ingredients thoroughly. Preheat your grill to low heat and grease the grates. Layer the vegetables grill for 12 minutes per side, until tender flipping once. Brush with the marinade/ dressing ingredients

Grilled Edamame Beans and Summer Squash

Ingredients

20 pcs. Edamame Beans

1 bunch of Romaine Lettuce leaves

1 summer squash, peeled and sliced lengthwise

4 large Tomatoes, sliced thick

Dressing Ingredients:

6 tbsp. extra virgin olive oil

1 tsp. onion powder

Sea salt, to taste 3 tbsp.

distilled white vinegar 1 tsp.

Directions:

Dijon mustard

Combine all of the dressing ingredients thoroughly. Preheat your grill to low heat and grease the grates. Layer the vegetables grill for 12 minutes per side, until tender flipping once. Brush with the marinade/ dressing ingredients

www.ingramcontent.com/pod-product-compliance
Lightning Source LLC
Chambersburg PA
CBHW070734030426
42336CB00013B/1966